e amazing *50 Ways* thrilled with this emotional eating. ithout calories. *50* :ked with creative, unique, healthy, and lasting alternatives to munching away your emotions."

> —**Mark Hyman, MD**, director of the Cleveland Clinic
> Center for Functional Medicine and author of the
> #1 *New York Times* bestseller *The Blood Sugar Solution*

"*50 More Ways to Soothe Yourself Without Food* is a fantastic resource for anyone who has struggled with emotional, mindless, or chaotic eating. Susan Albers provides a collection of practical, science-based, and tried-and-true strategies for breaking unhealthy cycles and cultivating mindfulness. Written in an authoritative but supportive and encouraging voice, Susan provides wisdom, and the ability to find calm and comfort, while simultaneously developing a nourishing, enjoyable, and balanced relationship with food."

> —**Cynthia Sass, MPH, MA, RD, CSSD**, *New York*
> *Times* best-selling author, contributing nutrition
> editor for *HEALTH* magazine, and owner of Sass
> Consulting Services, Inc.

D0029153

"Susan Albers does it again with *50 More Ways to Soothe Yourself Without Food*. With a friendly demeanor and can-do spirit, Albers successfully guides anyone who struggles with emotional eating—and who hasn't?—to make realistic, sustainable changes in their diet and their life. Jam-packed with science-based advice and practical solutions, this book will prove to be an asset to anyone who wants to get healthier and happier."

    —Elisa Zied, MS, RDN, CDN, author of
      Younger Next Week

"Food—usually *unhealthy* food—often becomes a substitute for love or other emotional support. In her book *50 More Ways to Soothe Yourself Without Food*, esteemed author Susan Albers provides simple, effective strategies to break that addictive cycle and satisfy your emotional needs without food's potentially destructive grip."

    —JJ Virgin, celebrity nutrition and fitness expert,
      and author of the *New York Times* bestsellers
      The Virgin Diet and *The Sugar Impact Diet*

"Why is it so hard to stop stress eating? Albers provides the key answers and reveals the root causes of emotional eating in her book *50 More Ways to Soothe Yourself Without Food*. This easy-to-read, fun, helpful guide will equip readers with the necessary tools to end emotional eating right now!"

> —**Sara Gottfried, MD**, *New York Times*
> best-selling author of *The Hormone Reset*
> *Diet* and *The Hormone Cure*

"I'm a big fan of Susan Albers. This book goes far beyond giving you tips and tricks to soothe yourself to curb emotional eating. This book gives you the essentials to live a fuller, healthier, and happier life. Really love this book!"

> —**Elisha Goldstein, PhD**, cofounder of
> the Center for Mindful Living and author
> of *Uncovering Happiness*

"Susan Albers's book, *50 More Ways to Soothe Yourself Without Food*, is brilliant! If you know what to eat, but can't manage to follow that advice, then you likely struggle with using food to soothe your stress. This very important book gives you practical and easy-to-follow tools to overcome emotional eating and optimize your health for a lifetime."

—**Steven Masley, MD**, best-selling author of *The 30-Day Heart Tune-Up*

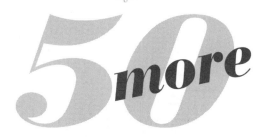

50 more

ways to
soothe yourself
without
food

Susan Albers, PsyD

New Harbinger Publications, Inc.

Publisher's Note

This publication is designed to provide accurate and authoritative information in regard to the subject matter covered. It is sold with the understanding that the publisher is not engaged in rendering psychological, financial, legal, or other professional services. If expert assistance or counseling is needed, the services of a competent professional should be sought.

Distributed in Canada by Raincoast Books

Copyright © 2015 by Susan Albers
New Harbinger Publications, Inc.
5674 Shattuck Avenue
Oakland, CA 94609
www.newharbinger.com

Cover design by Amy Shoup
Acquired by Catharine Meyers
Edited by Marisa Solís

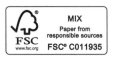

Library of Congress Cataloging-in-Publication Data

Albers, Susan.
  50 more ways to soothe yourself without food : mindfulness strategies to cope with stress and end emotional eating / Susan Albers.
      pages cm
  Includes bibliographical references.
  ISBN 978-1-62625-252-3 (paperback) -- ISBN 978-1-62625-253-0 (pdf e-book) --
ISBN 978-1-62625-254-7 (epub) 1. Stress (Psychology) 2. Eating disorders--Psychological aspects. 3. Food habits--Psychological aspects. I. Title. II. Title: Fifty more ways to soothe yourself without food.
  BF575.S75A4193 2015
  616.85'26--dc23
                                        2015030059

Printed in the United States of America

17   16   15

10   9   8   7   6   5   4   3   2   1   First printing

Dedicated to Brooklyn & Jack

Get inspired to start eating more mindfully today!

For a **free download** of the 20 best motivational quotes, visit http://www.eatingmindfully.com/motivation.

Contents

Mindful Eating Manifesto

Being nourished and well fed is critical to being at your best—to focus, create, innovate, authentically connect, and simply be the most amazing you. The first step to healthy eating is to focus more on *how* you eat than *what* you eat. It's perfectly okay to enjoy delicious food in a mindful way. When prepared well, healthy food is stunningly delicious and filling to the belly, and it exposes "junk food" as the highly processed stuff, pumped with artificial fluff, that it is. The comfort food brings is disappointingly fleeting. Hunger can be deceptive, and mindfulness can help distinguish emotional from true physical hunger. Whether you eat, snack, munch, dine, or take just one bite, always, always keep your mindful inner light switched on.

—Susan Albers, PsyD

Dear Reader,

Hi, I'm Susan Albers. It's a pleasure to meet you! I would like to congratulate you on the purchase of this book. It shows that you are interested in a healthy lifestyle and finding creative, effective ways to calm and comfort yourself without food. I'm a licensed clinical psychologist and a *New York Times* best-selling author who has, for more than eleven years, worked at one of the top five medical centers in the country. It is an honor to work at this internationally renowned institution helping people each day! I work with clients who struggle with emotional eating and stress eating on a daily basis. My clients come from all walks of life, from university professors and CEOs to stay-at-home moms and farmers. And no matter where they are in life or where they work or live, my clients overwhelmingly share many of the same emotional eating triggers.

Eating Mindfully, my first book on mindful and emotional eating, was published more than ten years ago, and an updated edition containing the latest mindful eating research was published last year. If you didn't realize it, the book you have in your hands is a sequel. It was written as a follow-up to my previous book, *50 Ways to Soothe Yourself Without Food*, because people from all over the world wrote to me and professed how life-changing the techniques have been. The book not only guided readers to end comfort eating, it also helped them to stop smoking and end other habits like chewing on their nails, to have better relationships, and to enjoy life more. Since that book, I've compiled fifty *more* ways to soothe yourself without eating; my efforts are now in your hands.

Sometimes people ask why I haven't become a full-time writer (this is my seventh book!). I shake my head emphatically, no. It's working with people directly that allows me to write in the first place! I continue to learn every single day about healthy, mindful eating from my clients and readers who talk to me in session or send me stories by e-mail.

Helping people one-on-one is one of my greatest joys. I get a candid glance into the real struggles people have with food—not made or manufactured ones but honest, real-life struggles. So if you have a story or insight about mindful eating or emotional eating, please send it to me! I'd like to help.

I have also gained valuable insight into emotional eating from my own family. I grew up in suburban Ohio, and to say that my Italian family loved to eat would be an understatement. They *loved* to eat! For every holiday, the Italian side would get together and decide the menu first, even before they would choose the date and time. It was *Food = Love*. To this day, my mom never shows up at my house without a grocery bag full of food and a menu planned for her stay. I'm not complaining! I just want to give you a picture of how large a role food can play in an extended family culture.

Interestingly, my father's side has a very different relationship to food. My grandparents were hard-working farmers of German descent who used every bit of food they grew on their Ohio farm. Their relationship to food was practical and varied by how well the crops and livestock were doing. The main question they had to answer each day was this: "What can I eat that will keep me filled until I am done plowing the fields?" My grandmother's handwritten cookbook was filled with recipes based only on the ingredients they had readily available on the farm—not what sounded delicious and yummy. To this day, my dad still thinks about food as fuel to power his workday—that's it.

What kind of family do you have? Is it a family with a practical relationship to food or one that has an emotional connection to what is eaten? Perhaps they spend a lot of time together going out to dinner, baking holiday cookies, eating birthday cake, or making favorite dishes. If so, you know what a challenge it is to unravel your emotional connection to food. It's likely been with you since you were born and may be unconsciously woven into your everyday life. But, it *is* possible to break that emotional connection! You can start being mindful of the influences your early family life has on your current food decision making and learn better ways to soothe yourself. If there is one thing that I've learned from my clients and family, it's this: ending emotional eating is *not* easy without a plan.

I am sensitive to the challenges of working full-time and taking care of a family, juggling an incredibly full personal life and career. I know that even mundane errands like picking up groceries, stopping at the bank, dropping off kids, paying bills, and getting to work on time can make your stress level sky-rocket. It is extraordinarily difficult, particularly for busy women and men, to find the time to take care of themselves. My clients often tell me that they come last on the list of people to take care of, after kids and partners—if they even put themselves on the list. I keep these challenges (exhaustion, feeling overworked, little time to yourself, and so on) in mind whenever I am sharing a technique. This book assumes that you don't have a full-time nanny, a personal chef, an assistant, and unlimited funds—all of which would help most people's stress level a bit!

As for me, I live and breathe the tools and techniques in *50 More Ways to Soothe Yourself Without Food*. If you followed me around for a day, you'd see that I typically use at least one technique a day, often more than that. Thankfully, for me, certain comfort foods still taste good, but they lost their power to calm me a long time ago—and the same is true for many of my clients. There are many other things that don't involve food that I now find soothing and look forward to. Yes, it was hard to get to a place where pasta and cookies don't have power over me. I've learned how to self-soothe without food, and I'll share these techniques with you as we go on this journey together.

Of course, it didn't happen overnight, but the good news is that it *did* happen and it *can* happen to you! I am going to show you how to rewire your brain so you too can stop finding eating soothing and start experiencing other ways to calm yourself, feel balanced, and be more in charge of your emotions. Keep in mind, there is a time and place for all of these techniques. The trick is learning what works best for you. We will explore that and more throughout these chapters. Thank you for inviting me on your journey—here we go!

Mindfully yours,
Susan Albers, PsyD

PART I

All About Emotional Eating

How It Happens

Think of a time when you were infatuated with someone. This person was all you could think about. Maybe you spent a lot of time daydreaming about him, doodling his name on a pad of paper. You think you might be falling in love. But then you go on your first date, and the wind deflates from your sails. For whatever reason, you realize he's not right for you and he never was what he seemed. In these tough moments, we experience the initial thrill of dating quickly followed by a huge letdown.

Perhaps you've had the same experience with food. You spend a lot of time thinking about, dreaming about, pining for, and imagining good eats. But then once you have them, they don't always deliver what you had hoped. Your fantasy of how it would make you feel is much different than how you actually feel. Food has let you down.

Let's hear from Melanie and her recent new relationship to food:

Life was good until I got a new boss. Every time she walked down the hallway, I'd cringe. I'd imagine Darth Vader–like music playing as she approached my desk. I found myself hiding behind my computer screen nibbling on candy and snacks; ninety-five percent of the time I wasn't even hungry. At home, I'd spend the night in front of the TV trying to shake off the stress from the day and unwind. Inevitably, I'd be mindlessly munching on a bowl of chips. When that was gone, I'd rummage around for something sweet. I tried many things to quit this habit: distracting myself, telling myself to just cut it out. These things worked for a little while. Then I needed something more. I realized that I had gained more than ten pounds in a year and a half. I believe it was 100 percent stress related.

If Melanie's story sounds familiar, you aren't alone. If you've picked up this book, it's likely that you too are well versed in comfort eating—eating to feel better. Like Melanie, emotional eating may have snuck up on you. Many of us instantly and automatically reach for food in moments of stress, anxiety, boredom, grief, happiness, heartache, and so on.

Why do we turn to food? There are many reasons that I will explain throughout this book. But the main motivation is that it offers *some* degree of relief from daily stress and tension. Eating a cookie or piece of cake can feel like waving a magic wand to poof away discomfort and anxiety. Within a matter of moments of biting into a chocolate bar, you can feel your anxiety level drop down from an 8 to a 4. Instant bliss. Some people drink alcohol, some take drugs, others go shopping. We eat. The sheer fact of the matter is that comfort eating works particularly when you want or *need* to feel better *right now*. Food is around us 24/7. The convenience factor plus instant gratification makes the perfect recipe for emotional eating.

So what's the problem? The moment of bliss is fleeting. It's clear in Melanie's story that the solution becomes another problem. Ask anyone just a few minutes after stress eating how she feels, and the story isn't pretty. What does she say? The list is long and often filled with regret: guilty, bloated, frustrated. The emotional 180 is intense. Sometimes people even feel angry. One of my clients says, "How could I let myself be seduced into comfort eating again? I know it doesn't make me feel good after the fact, and yet I do it over and over and over again!" This may be perplexing to you as well. Why do we continue to do something that ultimately doesn't work in the long run?

This is a mystery that I hope to solve for Melanie and for you too. Since I'm a psychologist who works with comfort eaters daily in my office, I recognize it immediately when I see it. Melanie had stepped onto what I frequently call the *Comfort Eating Carousel*. It's a cycle that goes like this:

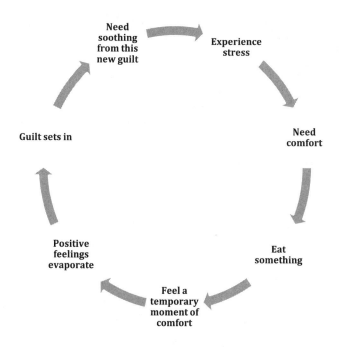

It's carousel-like because it keeps going around and around. You can get off, but you have to decide it's time. And it can be very tempting to hop back on and say, "Just one more ride!"

Most of my clients don't worry too much about emotional eating—at first. Little bits of it here and there are often no big deal. But when emotional eating becomes your go-to method for coping with stress, your quality of life begins to plummet. Sometimes this includes weight gain, feeling frustrated, becoming upset with yourself, or isolating yourself because you are embarrassed or uncomfortable in your body.

As you read this book, you will notice a couple of terms that I use frequently: *comfort eating* and *emotional eating*. These are both the same thing and may be used interchangeably to refer to eating that is related to emotion in one way or another. It is the use of food to lessen or avoid bad feelings, or to prolong good feelings. A subset of emotional eating is *stress eating*, which has the component of triggering a biological mechanism called the *HPA axis* (hypothalamic, pituitary, adrenal partnership). This axis controls your stress hormones and kicks your sympathetic nervous system into gear. It's this system that is biologically wired to make you crave sugary, fatty foods. All stress eating can be considered emotional or comfort eating, but not all emotional and comfort eating is stress eating.

It's likely that, if you're reading this, comfort eating is no longer working for you. You may have realized that eating is a temporary Band-Aid—it doesn't feel good or provide relief in the long run, and sometimes the post-eating feelings are worse than the initial ones. Perhaps, like Melanie, you've tried many things to put a stop to emotional eating. Some things may have worked for a while, but then you find that you are right back to doing it again. That is exactly where Melanie was when she walked into my office. She felt frustrated and stuck. She wanted some techniques to help her get off of the Comfort Eating Carousel.

If you're seeking answers and some skills to halt the cyclical habit, you're in the perfect place. In this book, you will find many exciting and innovative techniques. Some will be familiar to you and others will be brand new. Here's a snapshot of what this book offers:

- A thorough explanation of the reasons Melanie—and you!—fall into the trap of comfort eating time and again

- An examination of how emotional eating works and why it's so comforting in the moment

- Proven strategies for how to conquer emotional eating once and for all

- Real-life examples of replacing emotional eating with healthier activities

All of the techniques I discuss in my books and articles, and on blogs and my website, can be described in three ways: easy, economical, and effective.

Easy: It's important that any tip I share is simple. My tips are things that don't require a lot of time and can be done right *now*. They will not take you weeks and weeks to learn. And they aren't a struggle. They might take practice, but they'll result in less sweat and fewer tears.

Economical: The tips are easily affordable for anyone. The majority of my tips don't cost any money. Some may require a few supplies, but even those have a low price.

Effective: The techniques I share work! However, you don't have to take my word for it. They are all research-based tools. Therefore, although you may not have heard of some of these techniques, others have studied, researched, and implemented them. Their limitations will also be discussed.

How to Get the Most Benefit from This Book

This book has been created to function like a guidebook with a set of instructions that you can use whenever you need to. Keep this guide in your purse, briefcase, car, or on the coffee table and flip through it whenever you need ideas to stop emotional eating in its tracks.

It's helpful to start at the beginning of this book. You may be tempted to flip through the pages right off the bat, looking for chapters that appeal to you. But it's advisable to start by understanding a little bit about why emotional eating happens and where it comes from. This gives your mind the opportunity to understand the big picture.

Next, read through the entire book. Keep an open mind. As you read, you are likely to say, "Wow! That sounds just like me," or "I'm not sure that would work for me." Take notes. Jot down the strategies that you'd like to try. But don't give up on the ones you're unsure about—you might find the solution you've been hoping for!

Who This Book Is For

This book is for *anyone* who has ever struggled with emotional eating. In a nutshell, that is almost everyone. I'd like to meet someone who has not experienced emotional eating. (I have not met anyone yet—have you?)

It is also a book for men and women. While most of the examples may be of women (this is because the majority of my clients are female), I want to acknowledge that men emotionally eat as well (Macht, Roth, and Ellgring 2002). I've worked with men in my office, and many male readers tell me about the ways the messages in this book resonate with them. So don't hesitate to share this book with any friends who may be struggling too.

Now, let's go ahead and get off the Comfort Eating Carousel!

All About Emotional Eating and Self-Soothing

Think about a time you went home for the holidays. Your aunts, uncles, grandparents, and anyone else who is important to you are there around the table. When you first walk in the door, you instantly feel comforted by the warm, glowing feeling you get. The smell of the foods from the kitchen and the sounds of your family are familiar and comfortable. You feel connected and calm. Then, all of a sudden, one of your relatives asks you a nosy question about your relationship or your financial situation, and you become uncomfortable. Maybe two family members start the same argument they always have, perhaps another member of your family gets on your nerves with her strange mannerisms. Maybe the kids misbehave or someone eats the last piece of pie—the one you were dying to try. All of these little things add up. Now you feel regret for coming, and all you want to do is get out of there quickly.

This family scenario may mimic your feelings about food. You may want to keep this metaphor in mind when you consider how quickly emotional eating can make a 180 from pleasure to remorse. First, your senses are comforted and calmed by the familiar sensations. Warm and gooey, sweet and savory, salty and crunchy. But slowly, when boundaries are broken and your desire to stop eating isn't honored, the wonderful sensations you were just experiencing feel toxic.

The good news is that you can prevent your family and food from making the flip from comforting to noxious by being more mindful of your feelings and responding to them in the right way—in other words, by setting boundaries and finding ways to calm and comfort yourself without eating. Often, we try to force it. Your family or food was once really comforting when you were twelve, and you want that experience again. But you're older, and things aren't like that anymore; you keep trying to make the situation give you the feeling it once did.

Here is the main take-home message that I want you to get from this book: *Overeating is not a problem about food—it's a problem of self-soothing.* In other words, the issue we are really looking at is finding ways to calm down, de-stress, feel better, and get a grip. It's not only about fighting off food cravings for potato chips and cheese puffs. It's unrealistic to expect that you will throw away or avoid all the yummy food you crave in the world. Instead, it's important to be able to cope with cravings wherever and whenever they pop up. When you're able to manage your emotions, you no longer *need* to turn to food to feel better.

The problem is that, from an early age, few of us are taught self-soothing skills. It's unfortunate. We need them! Think of a baby in a crib who wakes in the middle of the night. At first the baby cries looking for some comfort, but eventually, with time and patient parents, the baby learns to self-soothe. Perhaps he sucks a pacifier, clings to his blankie, or rolls over.

Life is incredibly stressful. Has anyone ever sat you down and said, "Here is a lesson on how to deal with stress"? Or have you ever taken a class on how to manage difficult emotions and ways to self-soothe? No! We learn how to cope with stress in a variety of ways, mostly by watching other people. Maybe you calm down the same way your mother does. Or maybe you came across a solution by chance; for example, perhaps you noticed that playing a game on your phone helps you to de-stress for a moment, so you start to do it more often. Some self-soothing skills are very healthy (sleep, call a friend to vent, take a walk). Others are not (smoke, have a cocktail, eat). Think for a moment. How do you calm down after an argument with a friend or loved one? Unfortunately, sometimes self-soothing skills can be downright harmful (taking drugs, cutting).

Occasionally, comfort eating can develop into a more significant issue. Binge eating disorder has recently been accepted as an "official" diagnosis. It has been added to the *Diagnostic and Statistical Manual of Mental Disorders* (*DSM-5*), the big, universally accepted book of psychiatric disorders that doctors help use to diagnose patients. This is good news and a game changer. Why? It recognizes and pays homage to several things. First, there is a difference between overeating and eating triggered by emotions. Overeating is eating too large of a portion size because the food is there, or because you are unaware of how much is healthy for you to consume. Emotional and binge eating are prompted by emotions. Everyone falls somewhere on the spectrum from never emotionally eating to frequently eating because they are happy, sad, angry, or upset.

Examples of Self-Soothing

This is a brief list of some common feelings, behaviors, and thoughts comfort eaters have surrounding food. There are many other examples. Take a moment and see if any of these sound familiar to you.

Emotional Eating: Feelings

- Eating numbs my emotions.

- The urge to eat is triggered when I want to celebrate.

- I feel relief while eating.

- I feel empty, so I eat to feel more fulfilled.

- I have feelings of guilt post-eating.

Emotional Eating: Behaviors

- Chewing feels good.

- I rummage through cupboards seeking something specific to eat, but I have difficulty finding just what I want.

- Eating right away after a stressful event is a habit.

- I stock up on comfort foods in case I "need" them.

- Overeating at stressful events like holidays or family reunions is common.

- I'm searching for something to eat but can't find anything truly satisfying.

Emotional Eating: Thoughts

- I'll just continue to eat different foods because I can't find what I really want.

- I believe that eating = relaxing.

- When upset, I think, "I need to eat something."

- I focus only on particular types of foods for emotional relief, like chocolate, ice cream, chips, and so on.

- I think about eating so much that I'm hungry right after I've eaten.

- I know that I am only eating this food because I am stressed.

Integrative Medicine: Going Beyond

Many of the techniques in this book are based on the field of *integrative medicine*, a more modern term for what used to be known as *complementary and alternative medicine* (CAM). This reflects the integration of "alternative" treatments with conventional medicine and research. Those interested in this field tend to shy away from the word "alternative," because it implies that a treatment is not generally accepted or is off the map in some way, when many of the techniques are not. To date, most people are more familiar with the term "alternative." But, throughout this book, you will see both terms.

CAM is traditionally thought of as practices rooted in ancient traditions that are often not in the core curriculum taught in medical school. That said, the popularity of these techniques is on the rise; they're starting to be a part of many medical programs and are being tested in clinical research. The treatments are often an adjunct or addition to typical therapies. Sometimes they even replace them. At the core of these techniques is the belief that the body is powerful and can be involved in healing itself. The good news, and something that is important to me as a therapist and clinician, is that the efficacy of many of these techniques has been researched and reported on in published journals. Several national surveys estimate that almost 40 percent of the U.S. population uses complementary and alternative medicine therapy in a given year (Gray et al. 2002). One large mail survey (Gray et al. 2002) found that the most commonly used techniques were relaxation (18 percent), massage (12 percent), herbal medicine (10 percent), or megavitamin therapy (9 percent).

What does this mean? You might already be included in this group. If you've done deep breathing exercises or yoga, you've used alternative or complementary medicine. Maybe you've put honey in tea to soothe your throat when it was sore or drank warm milk to help you sleep—also CAM. My grandmother was an advocate of CAM techniques—although she called them "home remedies." She believed they were natural, less expensive, and, for certain ailments, more effective. For example, when I got a sunburn as a child (the days before SPF 50) she didn't reach for a cooling spray to help alleviate the pain; my grandmother went to her windowsill and snapped off the end of an aloe vera plant, then rubbed the comforting, gentle substance on my burn.

To this day, I make sure I have an aloe vera plant somewhere in my house for just that occasion. My guess is that you use some CAM techniques as well, whether you're aware of it or not.

Some of the skills in this book may be less familiar to you, such as *mindfulness techniques* or the use of *expressive arts therapies*. If so, that is okay, they will be explained in full.

Why would we turn to these types of techniques? Different things work for different people. Why not try *everything* that might work? Here is a list of reasons people have for turning to integrative or CAM techniques:

- You don't want to take medication.

- There is no Western medication or effective therapy that is available.

- You feel stuck. You tried other techniques and they don't seem to be working.

- You're bored. You want to try something new.

- Nothing is working. You feel frustrated.

- New circumstances bring on the need for more tools to choose from.

- Your personality is nontraditional. You don't like conventional treatments.

- You feel that your issue is more mental than physical, and you know that medication isn't going to get rid of situational stress.

- You need something that doesn't cost a lot of money.

- You want a skill you can practice anywhere, anytime, whenever your emotions or symptoms hit.

- You want a healing modality that recognizes you as a complete human being—body, mind, and spirit—not just a symptom.

The Goal: Calm, Cool, Collected, Comforted

Let me explain what you can and cannot expect from CAM techniques. CAM techniques are not a magic wand. So unfortunately they won't go "poof" and take away all your urges for comfort eating. And they won't eliminate *all* bad feelings or discomfort. The goal isn't to turn off your feelings or make them vanish—although sometimes you might love to make that happen. Instead, the intention is to cool them off or turn them down so they don't push you to food for immediate relief. When you are able to manage and cope with your feelings, you can then create and choose healthier options. Life would be boring if all your feelings were erased. Also, emotions help you to make decisions. So, let *calm, cool, collected, and comforted* be your motto and mantra.

The purpose of CAM and integrative methods is not to induce a joyous or elated feeling, although sometimes this happens. The outcome we can hope to access is comfort and ease.

Here is my disclaimer: If you struggle with an eating disorder, or if you have tried the techniques in this book and aren't getting anywhere, it is vitally important that you contact a professional such as a licensed therapist, physician, or dietitian. If you have any medical or physical limitations, only participate in activities that your doctor or health care practitioner approves of. This is essential. If you are not sure about a technique, simply give him or her a call and ask. Fortunately, these tools can be an adjunct to or complement what you are already doing, even if it is traditional medicine.

Emotional Eating: Why We Do It

What happens if you don't address emotional eating and keep riding the Comfort Eating Carousel? Maybe you turned a blind eye for a while or chose to put it on a shelf until you were able to cope with it, or until your life "settled down." If you are an emotional eater, it's likely that you already know what can happen by ignoring it. In the short term, nothing; life continues as usual. In the long run, emotional eating that becomes your main way of coping becomes problematic. Emotional eaters often develop minor and major health and physical problems. Minor issues include frustration, weight gain, difficulty fitting into your clothing, spending too much money on snacks and junk food, eating unhealthily, self-consciousness, remorse, and guilt. If left unchecked, emotional eating has the potential to spiral into type

2 diabetes, eating disorders, depression, heart disease, and so on. The point is that it's important to take a good, hard look at your emotional eating to prevent it from mounting into something more serious. Or if emotional eating is already in full swing, learning techniques to stop it in its tracks will help mitigate or eliminate some of the physical and mental effects.

Learning to Self-Soothe the Right Way

The need to self-soothe, or regulate our feelings, starts from day one, when you are born. When a baby cries, he or she has to find a way to settle down. Some babies are wired in a way that they settle down quite easily, even on their own. Others need help by being rocked, held, or talked to.

Your caregivers played an important role in teaching you self-soothing skills, and you internalized the way they help to calm you down. For example, my own mother always says, "Try, and try again." It's like her personal mantra. I notice that I say these words to myself whenever something doesn't work out quite right or I've made a mistake. Saying this to myself helps to ease the disappointment and encourages me to try again, even when I don't feel like it. I learned this from my mom.

You also learn a lot from the other people in your life— mostly through observing what they do. Sometimes you take on or "model" the way they calm themselves down.

You can often spot a person who doesn't have strong self-soothing skills or doesn't practice them when stressed. Small things can very easily upset them. Also, they have difficulty talking themselves through problems rationally, get stuck brooding or dwelling, have difficulty letting things go, or seek something outside of themselves (drugs, alcohol, food) to feel better. For example, maybe you've met someone who has fallen to pieces over a frustrating event like waiting in line. Imagine this scene for a moment. The checkout person realizes that an item doesn't have a price tag and calls for someone to get the price. The line comes to a standstill. Some people in line will say to themselves, "Oh well, this happens." They may look at magazines or their phone to distract themselves and pass the time. The person without self-soothing skills may start to get upset, tap his or her foot loudly, make comments, or worse.

If you don't have strong self-soothing skills, that's okay! The purpose of this book is to teach them to you!

But Why Does Eating Feel So Darn Good?

Let's hear from Mandy, one of my clients:

> At first I didn't think that emotional eating was a big deal. I rationalized that I was going through a lot; it was what I needed to cope. I had just gotten a divorce and

moved back home to take care of my aging parents, and my children had gone off to college. One day I stepped on the scale and realized I had gained thirty pounds in one year! I was so depressed. I felt like my quality of life had plummeted.

In the absence of strong self-soothing skills, it's easy to turn to food to help manage feelings. It is a cheap, legal, readily accessible option. Yes, we know that food is soothing and comforting, and that we eat when we are feeling certain emotions. But why? It may be more complex than you think.

Common Reasons for Emotionally Eating

Let's review some of the most common reasons we turn to food when we need an emotional fix:

- **The feel-good fix:** Eating doesn't just feel good because of the sensory pleasure to our tongues (although that is part of it). There are chemicals at work when we eat. It's important to realize that food often changes our neurochemistry. Good food, for example, stimulates *dopamine*, a neurotransmitter that regulates pleasure. When researchers test the brain response of people who are overweight, they often find that the pleasure center of their brain lights up more intensely than others (Weltens, Zhao, and Van Oudenhove 2014). What does that mean? It means that, for certain people, food just doesn't taste good; it gives an extreme amount of pleasure. Eating has also been linked to changes in *serotonin level*, which is also boosted by taking antidepressants (Young 2007). In many ways, you could say eating is like taking a food antidepressant for some!

- **Stress and an effort to rebalance:** We tend to eat more when we feel stressed out. In part, it's due to the stimulation of the *HPA axis* (hypothalamus, pituitary gland, and adrenal glands), which is triggered when you feel overwhelmed. Your body becomes flooded with *cortisol*, the hormone that makes you crave sugary, fatty, calorie-dense foods. There are biological reasons for this. In caveman times, when you were stressed you needed all the energy you could muster to fight off the threat (think lion). Now you are no longer faced with lions, but smaller things cause your system to click into a stressed-out mode nevertheless. Studies show that increases in cortisol predict an increase in body mass (Roberts, Campbell, and Troop 2014). That means, when stressed, people work less to restrict their eating and are driven to eat to feel better. It explains why we often crave good food when feeling overwhelmed by a work project or the constant audible alerts of a mobile phone.

- **More, please!** Eating prolongs positive feelings and sometimes elevates them. If you feel happy, sometimes food makes you feel even happier and for a longer period of time. It's a myth that we only eat emotionally when we are sad. In fact, studies show what happy people like to munch on most—pizza, steak, and popcorn are favorites (Wansink, Cheney, and Chan 2003).

- **Accessibility!** Let's face it. Comfort foods are everywhere. It's hard to escape them. We often have access to sugary, fatty food 24/7. The convenience factor makes it an attractive way to calm and soothe ourselves. It's easy—sometimes too easy!

- **Media diet:** We often turn to comfort foods when stressed because of what we expect to happen, based on the media and ads, which often link foods with certain emotions. Think about chocolate ads, for example. They're often tied to words like "bliss," "relaxing," "you deserve it," "escape," and so on. When these foods and words are paired repeatedly, people begin to expect these emotions to follow after eating. One of the best examples of this relates to a woman's menstrual cycle. Numerous TV shows, ads, and pop culture suggest that women crave chocolate during their period. Research actually indicates otherwise (McVay et al. 2012)! To date, there is no known clear biological reason for craving chocolate during menstruation. Society suggests that women expect to crave it; therefore they do.

- **Thumb twiddling:** Sometimes people eat out of sheer boredom. You don't know what else to do, and eating fills a block of time. One of the things that you will learn in this book is how to be okay with downtime. Giving yourself permission to have free spaces of time without doing something, and learning how to tolerate boredom, is important. This isn't always easy, but it's essential if you are going to kick the boredom-eating habit.

- **Habit:** A significant portion of emotional eating is nothing more than habit. You do it, like brushing your teeth or your hair, because it's what you always do. It's part of a routine. The good news is that you can break or rework habits. They aren't set in stone. So if you suspect that you comfort eat out of mere habit, we can change that!

- **Distraction:** One theory is that eating distracts from emotions (Polivy and Herman 1999). When you're eating, you're focusing your mind in a different direction. Instead of dealing with how upset, angry, tearful, hurt, or fearful you are, you eat.

- **Ignoring internal cues:** When stressed, sometimes people become insensitive to their internal cues of hunger and fullness. As a result, you confuse emotional arousal (an increase of feelings) as hunger. So if you're not tuned in to your internal cues, you're more vulnerable to eating when stressed without even realizing it.

- **Alexithymia:** The condition in which people have difficulty putting their feelings into words is called *alexithymia*. The more trouble you have talking about or expressing your feelings, the more likely you are to emotionally eat (Pinaquy et al. 2003).

- **Impulsivity:** You simply don't stop to consider decisions fully but impulsively grab for something to put in your mouth without thinking about it.

Self-Soothing Reflection

Now that you know the reasons that people engage in emotional eating, take a moment to answer the following two questions. Write your answers down in a journal so you can reflect on them later.

- Which of the reasons listed on the previous pages describe why I engage in emotional eating, comfort eating, or stress eating?

- What do I gain emotionally from comforting eating? (Perhaps relief, a sense of calm, happiness, entertainment?)

Where to Go from Here

As you've learned from this chapter, food is soothing! You wouldn't overeat if it didn't work to calm you down and make you feel better. The good news is that there are other activities and strategies that will make you feel okay but won't lead to weight gain, regret, or guilt. Before we get to them, however, there are a few more things very much worth knowing.

15 Things You Didn't Know About Emotional Eating

Here are some interesting facts I've discovered in my research on comfort eating:

You only get a three-minute fix. A study reported in the journal *Appetite* gave participants chocolate and tested how long the "feel good" feeling lasts. It turns out that comfort and bliss only last three minutes (Macht and Mueller 2007). *Three minutes!* Isn't it a surprise how short-lived comfort eating can be?

Cake plus guilt equals less weight loss. Cake is a comfort food that can be associated with guilt and worry or pleasure and enjoyment. In a study of dieters, those who associated cake with "guilt" as opposed to "celebration" were less likely to lose weight over a three-month period. Those who had positive feelings and associated cake with being a comfort food were more likely to lose weight during those three months (Kuijer and Boyce 2014). The take-home message: guilt can derail your efforts.

Comfort foods are not cross-cultural. Have you assumed that chocolate is the go-to feel-better food everywhere in the world? It's not. People in different countries find comfort from various foods. For example, in Japan, miso soup, *okayu* (rice porridge that is made when children are sick), and ramen are popular comfort foods. In India, it's samosas, potato-stuffed crisps served with spicy green chutney. In Italy, it's ribbons of fresh pasta or potato gnocchi. When I was visiting Japan, my host family was appalled by the supersweet chocolate I brought for them to try. Their tongues were not used to it. This was clearly not one of their comfort foods—to my surprise!

There's a gender difference. According to one study (Wansink, Cheney, and Chan 2003), males prefer warm, hearty, meal-related comfort foods (such as steak, casseroles, and soup), while females prefer comfort foods that are more snack related (such as chocolate and ice cream).

We choose out of habit. When we're stressed out, we tend to revert back to the foods we frequently eat—whether they are healthy or not. A study presented at the Institute for Food Technologists Annual Meeting and Expo tested fifty-nine MBA students at the University of California during midterm exams. During peak stress times, students were more likely to choose the snacks they eat most frequently (Neal, Wood, and Drolet 2013). This is likely because it takes less thought and cognitive effort to choose familiar foods.

PMS doesn't trigger hormonal chocolate craving. Many people are under the misperception that hormonal changes make us crave chocolate during that time of the month. However, 80 percent of menopausal women still report chocolate cravings despite no longer having menstrual cycles or significant variability in their hormone levels during the course of a month (Hormes and Rozin 2009). The theory is that our desire for comfort and our stress about the approaching time of month causes us to turn to a culturally reinforced way of coping. In other words, we expect that chocolate will help, so we begin to crave it, not exactly because hormones are driving us to it.

Ritual is comforting. Do you eat comfort foods in a certain way? For example, do you eat the icing off your cupcake first or cut your peanut butter sandwich in half every time? Most of us have particular ways in which we eat food. A study published in the journal *Psychological Science* found that performing a ritual (like cutting a food in a particular way or eating it in a specific sequence) makes food taste better and gives you more enjoyment (Vohs et al. 2013). In this study, participants broke a chocolate bar in half without unwrapping it and ate it one half at a time. The nonritual group ate the chocolate however they wanted. Those who performed the ritual with the chocolate bar enjoyed it more.

It is not just the taste. We often think that comfort foods taste good because of the sensory experience against our lips and how the act of eating it *feels*. But in a study reported in the *Journal of Clinical Investigation*, researchers injected a fat-based solution right into the participants' stomachs that would cause a similar brain response to comfort foods. Then the researchers induced sadness. Functional MRI studies found that compared to the group that received an injection of saline solution, the people who got the fatty solution had a dampening of the part of the brain that responds to sadness. In other words, the ones with the fatty comfort food solution didn't feel as bad. Something biological is actually triggered in the stomach that sends signals to the brain to make us feel good (Van Oudenhove et al. 2011).

Happy people overeat too. Feeling good *and* bad triggers emotional eating. Yes! Even good feelings bring on the comfort-food craving. A study in the journal *Appetite* found that happier people are more likely to overeat compared to unhappy people (Bongers et al. 2013). It's a fact that isn't as well known.

Chicken soup can make you feel less lonely. Does chicken soup comfort you? If so, here's why: A study in *Psychological Science* found that people who ate chicken noodle soup felt less lonely while eating it and were able to come up with more relational words about their feelings while eating it (Troisi and Gabriel 2011). In other words, if you eat the soup while talking to someone, you are more successful in connecting with them. Comfort foods = comforting feelings = comfort around others.

Comfort is desired until the end. A study on death row inmates found that the last food requested by prisoners were calorie-dense comfort foods—67 percent chose fried foods, 66 percent picked desserts (Wansink, Kniffin, and Shimizu 2012). Honestly, is anyone surprised?

Familiar food can be comforting when away from home. A study of students studying abroad in England found that eating familiar comfort foods provided emotional substance (Edwards, Hartwell, and Brown 2010). Familiar food = comfort when away from home. (On the other hand, eating foods that are native to the land you are in, rather than your own, is a sign of being acculturated and integrated with your new environment, according to the researchers.)

Money shapes your perception of comfort foods. A recent study of participants in Canada found that people who are food secure—meaning they can routinely afford foods of their choice—describe Kraft Dinner (macaroni and cheese) as a comfort food. In contrast, people who are food insecure—meaning they experience an inability to obtain sufficient, nutritious, satisfying food choices, or uncertainty that they will be able to—do not describe Kraft Dinner as comfort food (Rock, McIntyre, and Rondeau 2009). Because it is an easy and inexpensive meal to prepare, it is often donated to food pantries and becomes a monotonous meal for those who use pantries, which does not produce positive feelings. In other words, a comfort food is one of choice, not necessity.

Dieters are the most prone to comfort eating. Researchers assert that the typical person drawn to emotional eating during chronic stress often tends to have a BMI (body mass index) above normal, a low mood, and high cortisol reactivity (high stress). This type of person tries to restrain his or her eating (Roberts et al. 2007). Interestingly, it is dieters who are most prone to emotional eating. Trying to restrain yourself actually backfires!

It's dose dependent. In one study by Macht and Mueller (2007), participants received only five grams of chocolate. This is approximately one-ninth of a regular-size Hershey's bar. This was not enough to lead to changes in mood. Unfortunately, very large quantities of food are often needed to make even a dent in your mood.

As you can see from this list, we know a lot about emotional eating, but we still have a long way to go. Every day, researchers are continuing to unravel the biological mechanisms (hormones, chemicals, etc.) that lead us to emotional eating. For now, let's lean more about what drives you to emotionally eat.

PART II

The Practices

Mindfulness Today

Many of my clients say that part of their stress and their difficulty making a healthy food decision is that their mind is cluttered with other things. When their minds jump from one thing to another, before they know it their hand is reaching into the cookie jar—and the cookie is gone before they give it a moment's thought. *Mindfulness* is keeping your mind focused and moving *with* a thought rather than trailing behind it.

A still and clear mind makes more thoughtful and discerning food decisions. It's when you lapse back into habit or are on autopilot that you click unconsciously into stress eating.

This part of the book will explore the many ways to leverage mindfulness when it comes to emotional eating, from mindful movement and speaking to mindful consumption and biofeedback. We will even explore how to use visualization and distraction as a means to bring yourself back to the present—for those times when being mindful seems impossible to do.

Let's begin with some ideas of ways you can be more mindful.

1. Learning How to "Be" More Mindful

Wayne Dyer has written in many of his books that we are called "human *beings*" for a reason: we are meant to simply be—or exist—rather than constantly feeling like our identities are tied to our actions and what we "do." He urges readers to realize that everyone is "good enough," and that there is nothing that you need to actively "do" to be good, worthy, and so on.

This directly relates to comfort eating, because when we feel bored, tired, lonely, or blue, we typically want to *act*, and that means we may start looking around for something to do: in this case, we want to eat. But instead of always "doing" something and asking ourselves, "What should I *do* now?" let's change that around and ask, "How should I *be*?"

"Being" means that you are just sitting with your feelings, allowing them to be whatever they are...until they eventually pass. Instead of trying to "do" something—like smother your feelings with brownies or distract yourself from thoughts by munching on chips—you can simply feel your feelings. Really experience them! You might say, "Heck yeah, I feel lonely right now. So what?" or "Of course I'm a little blue today, I know."

Yes, this can be scary at first, especially if food is your default mechanism for anything that feels uncomfortable. But trust yourself and the process. The feelings are just that—feelings. They won't do anything to you. So if you can just *exist* as you experience whatever feelings come up for you, know that eventually those emotions will pass. Over time, you may even find yourself being able to exist with your emotions with a sense of detachment: instead of judging yourself, your thoughts, and your feelings, you will be able to be an observer of them.

If you're new to being mindful, simply sitting with your emotions may seem too intimidating at first. If that is the case for you, try the following exercise to begin to become more mindful.

Soothing Strategy
Mentally SIT

Have you ever owned a new puppy? Puppies have a very short attention span. One minute they are totally enthralled in chasing a ball, and the next they hear a car door and make a beeline for the road. Their energy is uncontrolled and all over the place—one reason they require a lot of attention and training.

How do we try to rein in our own meandering attention span? Think of the command "Sit." The puppy is often able to sit for a moment and then goes bounding off again to the next thing. You call it back again and gently say, "Sit." You are forgiving rather than harsh toward the puppy because, hey, that's what puppies do—it's expected and part of their nature. Like the puppy, you can train your own mind to "sit" and "come back" to the task at hand.

When your mind is racing and begging for comfort food, tell yourself to mentally SIT and do the following meditation. When your mind wants to wander away, use the voice you would use for the puppy. Say to your mind, gently but firmly, "Sit." Don't let your thought run off to the next thing. Stay with it for just a moment. Take a breath. Be honest with yourself about how you are feeling.

You don't actually have to be sitting on a chair to do this exercise, though it works well that way. You can be lying down, standing, or even driving. Once in position, take just 1 minute to try this. Being very in tune with your current state of mind will help you to make the next food decision—mindfully—and steer you clear of emotional eating.

- **Stop.** Ask your mind to sit still for a moment, not run from place to place. What are you feeling right now? Pause your mind in this moment. How does your body feel? Are you emotionally or physically hungry?

- **Inspect.** Notice your thoughts nonjudgmentally. Don't judge your thoughts. Just observe them. Or try to be neutral about them. (For instance, say to yourself, "Oh, look, there is that thought again telling me that I can't stand it and that I must eat!")

- **Take a breath.** Re-center with a refreshing burst of oxygen to the brain. Say, "I am here in this moment."

Then, make an active decision. Is there another option (from this book!) that can help soothe your current mood?

Soothing Strategy
Shift into This Moment

If you find yourself struggling to stay present and calm, try this technique:

Shift into the present moment and connect with your senses. Pay attention to the sights, sounds, smells, feelings, and tastes that surround you. You may wish to do this by naming three things in front of you that you see, then identifying what you're hearing, and so on.

Next, touch your thumb to your index finger. As you do, say, "I am present."

Now, touch your thumb to your middle finger. As you do, say, "I am okay just as I am."

Then, touch your thumb to your ring finger. As you do, say, "I am calm."

Finally, touch your thumb to your little finger. As you do, say, "I am in charge of only this moment, not the next or the last."

As you complete this progression, notice yourself shift into the moment.

Soothing Strategy
"Squeegee Breath"

Have you ever used a squeegee on a car or kitchen window? Or maybe you've seen a professional window washer use one? In a sweeping motion, you can wipe a window clean in one stroke, leaving a shiny and clear pane of glass in its place.

Take what I call a "squeegee breath." Use this imagery when you need to let go of stress, worry, or irritation. Go ahead and give it a try now!

Take a deep breath. Focus on the top of your head.

As you exhale, imagine the stress escaping along with your breath. Visualize the squeegee going all the way from your head down to your toes.

Repeat 3 times.

Your vision will become clear only when you look into your heart. Who looks outside, dreams. Who looks inside, awakens.
—Carl Jung

2. Moving Mindfully

Sarah, my forty-two-year-old client, made tremendous strides in using mindful movement—bringing her attention to her body—to break free from what she called the "pitchfork folly." During one session, Sarah explained that, as a child, she worked on a farm in Ohio. Her job was to take care of horses. As she worked day after day, she went into a zone of mindlessly scooping and throwing the hay. Scoop. Throw. Scoop. Throw. Time flew by. One day, Sarah didn't even realize that there was nothing left to scoop; her pitchfork clanked loudly against the floor and the thud sent pain radiating up her shoulder. She never forgot that moment. It woke her up and thrust her expectantly back into her body. From that day forward, she paid attention to each time she thrust the fork down and to the way her muscles strained as she pulled up the hay and threw it into the air. It kept her mind from floating off.

Years later, the "pitchfork folly" popped up in her life again. Sarah noticed herself scooping up mac and cheese from a ceramic bowl in a rhythmic fashion. Scoop. Eat. Scoop. Eat. Before she knew what happened, the mac and cheese was gone, her spoon clanking against the bottom of the bowl. She hadn't even really enjoyed what she normally liked eating.

You may not be using a pitchfork, but you know what it is like to lock into autopilot with a fork, spoon, or even just your fingers. We've all experienced times when we are floating through our day, just flitting and fleeting from one thing to another, not really engaged or inhabiting our bodies. The risk? Your body slips into ingrained habits and takes it wherever it wants to go. It is often something outside of yourself that jolts you out of your mental fog.

The remedy to Sarah's autopilot actions? It was staying engaged with her body and being mindful of her movement. Whether Sarah is eating, walking, sleeping, working, or exercising, she stays present in her body. She makes a conscious effort to notice not only what her body is doing but what it is telling her by the way it moves. If she is slumped over her desk, she is tired. If she is balling up her fists, she is likely angry. When she feels confident, her heels click rather than shuffle. And when she eats, she is mindful of how her hands move, how her fingers grip the spoon, and how her arm brings the food up to her mouth.

Try it right now. Look down and notice how you are sitting. Are your legs crossed? Or are your feet flat on the ground. Is your back resting against the chair or is it angled forward? Are you sitting on a comfy, squishy pillow or is your bottom on a hard, wooden chair? Now, intentionally move your body in some way. Cross your legs in the opposite direction. Or roll your ankles around. Sit forward or back. Pay attention to how your body felt just a moment ago and how it feels now as you intentionally bring your attention to it. It's likely that you notice an interesting shift from feeling nothing in particular to noticing your body.

Paying attention to your body helps you become more attuned to the cues that your brain sends out with respect to when to stop and when to start eating. Your body does talk to you. I can't tell you how many clients have said to me, "I was so busy running around that I forgot to eat. When I stopped, I realized I was starving." Often, I tell these clients that they were likely hungry, but they didn't feel the hunger because they were tuned out of their body and focused on whatever they were thinking about. This leaves them at high risk to overeat when they do finally slow down, because their body is screaming, "Feed me!"

This kind of awareness is what allows you to differentiate real hunger from other emotions like boredom, irritation, or anxiety. You're actually tuned in to your body. You know how it feels, and you are the caretaker of its needs. This is when you and your body are on the same page. Believe me, I know that it is difficult to distinguish sometimes between emotional and physical hunger. A reader sent me an e-mail just this week that read, "I could eat a meal 24/7. I always feel hungry." It's likely that she is having extreme difficulty telling the difference between true hunger and an emotionally rooted craving. You may have times when you're disconnected from those feelings too. In these instances, you aren't paying attention to the subtleties—you're ignoring your body and brain signals. During these times, you may wish to use movement as a way of curbing your cravings and remaining mindful.

Two studies in the journal *Appetite* suggest that a short bout of exercise (for example, a fifteen-minute walk) can reduce chocolate cravings (Oh and Taylor 2013) as well as reduce spontaneous snacking on chocolate (Oh and Taylor 2012). What's more, walking with a positive attitude—upright posture, arms swinging at your sides—improves your mood and happiness level. Mood and body movement exert a mutual influence on each other. Walking briskly induces happiness and can lift depression, while curling up into the fetal position makes you feel like you have no control over your experiences and makes them more painful (Bohns and Wiltermuth 2011).

Bottom line? Movement has so many health benefits that when you get a craving—especially when you're not actually hungry—a brisk walk may be all you need to let it pass. But, tuning in mindfully while you move (see the following Soothing Strategy) gives you extra benefits.

Soothing Strategy
Craving a Walkabout

When you have a craving for chocolate (or any other yummy food), remember the study in the journal of *Appetite* mentioned previously. While simply just getting some exercise may hold the key to beating cravings, I challenge you to walk *mindfully*—not just to lace up your shoes and hit the pavement but to go for a *mindful* walk or run (which I'll describe shortly). Why? It's fantastic practice for honing your mindfulness skills. Not only is it scientifically proven to help you beat your cravings, it's a great opportunity to practice being in sync with your body and to sidestep emotional eating.

In addition to using movement to create an interruption of a craving, you can also move mindfully to induce relaxation. One welcome side effect of this is a reduced desire to eat emotionally, since your mindful movements will calm you.

Walking meditations are also wonderful ways to work out problems, reflect, sort out feelings, and focus on what's important. Anything that pops into your mind is fair game and fodder for your thought process. Just let the thoughts come in, swish around your mind, and float off. Oftentimes you'll think of solutions to problems, figure out how to do something better, or even reconcile your feelings more fully than you would at home on the sofa. Hopefully, you will begin to notice a pattern: More mindfulness, less unconscious eating. Greater relaxation, less tension. More presence, less guilt. Increased embracing of emotion, less temptation to use food to cover your true feelings.

Here is how you can approach a mindful walk or run:

- **Pay attention to your body.** As you begin to walk or jog, pay attention to your body as it moves. Notice the muscles that are working hard, like thighs, calves, and shoulders, for instance. How do they feel? Note any other sensations. Pay attention to the sound of your feet against the floor.

- **Be aware of your senses.** Notice the temperature of the air on your skin, the feeling of your clothes against your body, and the smells and sounds that surround you. Feel your footfall as you place one foot in front of the other.

Pay attention to the noises (cars, birds, other people, and so on), along with any other sensory experiences.

- **Notice your breath.** Is it shallow? Deep? Are you breathing through your nose or mouth? Is your breathing fast or slow? These questions will allow you to remain in tune with the present moment.

- **Acknowledge any discomfort.** If you begin feeling slight pain or pressure somewhere in your body—such as a cramp or sore muscle—try to stay with the feeling rather than trying to distract yourself. Sometimes this will allow your body to relax and release the pain more quickly than if you try to take your mind off of the uncomfortable feeling. (Of course, stop immediately and seek medical attention if the pain is severe, unusual, or puts you at risk for greater injury.)

If you are interested in going one step further, you can do this walking or running meditation regularly as yet another way to enhance well-being and promote relaxation. Both running and walking meditation involve focusing on your breath and letting any other thoughts that enter your mind simply pass through.

Soothing Strategy
Walking with Mindful Style

Now that you've gotten the hang of mindful walking from the previous strategy, try using different motions to unlock different feelings. Again, use walking as a vehicle for practicing this skill. There are lots of ways to walk—and many words to describe them—and the way you hold your body significantly impacts how you feel. Walk for 20 minutes using one of these styles. Notice whether the mood of your gait alters your feelings, even just a little. For instance, does skipping make you just a little happier?

Amble: an aimless walk

Bounce: with a spring

Skip: an energetic hop

Clump: heavily, as if weighted

Hike: long and purposeful

Limp, lumber, or lurch: slowly and heavily

March: rhythmically, in step

Mosey: without hurry

Pace: back and forth with drive

Parade: with fanfare

Plod: slowly, wearily

Pound: as if pounding the pavement

Prance: almost as if dancing

Sashay: with a sassy attitude

Stomp: to get out frustrations

Stroll: without a care in the world

Stride: like you own the block

Strut: like on a runway

Tiptoe: so that no one will notice you

Trample: with the attitude that it doesn't matter who sees you

Wander: as if it doesn't matter where

Words represent your intellect. The sound, gesture, and movement represent your feelings. —Patricia Fripp

3. Speaking Mindfully

Artist Vincent van Gogh once said, "If you hear a voice within you say, *you cannot paint,* then by all means paint, and that voice will be silenced." Sadly, it's all too easy for us to fall prey to negative conversations with ourselves.

You can't find your keys, and you think, "I always lose things!" Or a romantic relationship has come to an end and you tell yourself, "No wonder—I'm unlovable. I'll never find someone else." When left unchecked, this type of negative thinking can run amok, constantly replaying its harmful message in the back of your mind.

So why don't we stop already? It's so much easier said than done. Most of us know this isn't good for us, and it's no way to achieve anything positive. But if it's your go-to when times are tough, it may be a habit you're going to have to learn to break.

It's true that *positive self-talk* can be uplifting, inspirational, and motivating. When you congratulate yourself for a job well done or think, "I can do it!" these mental "conversations" often lead to positive outcomes and feelings. Unfortunately, many people fall victim to the opposite—*negative self-talk*—and constantly berate themselves for infractions both big and small, particularly around the way they eat. They then feel guilty, bitter, resentful, and depressed—which is a recipe for emotional eating.

One of the most convincing bodies of research on self-talk is linked to elite athletes. Time and again, when athletes use motivational ("You can do it!") and instructional ("Focus!") self-talk, there is great success. In a study of elite sprinters, the runners used self-talk with certain words at specific times: "push" when they needed to speed up, "heel" when they'd reached their ultimate speed, and "claw" to keep them going (Cutton and Hearon 2014). The athletes who used this technique ran faster— .26 seconds faster—which, for an elite athlete, can make all the difference between winning and losing.

As you listen to your own self-talk, consider whether it falls into one of three categories: self-evaluation ("I did that all wrong"), motivational ("You go, girl!"), or instructional ("One step at a time"). Many emotional eaters are stuck in the self-evaluation category and miss the benefits of motivational and instructional self-talk. Unfortunately, the more we beat ourselves up in our minds, the more often we will be tempted to eat for emotional reasons. To soothe that negative mental soundtrack, a heaping bowl of sweetened, sugary cereal or bag of tortilla chips could quell those feelings—at first. But the aftermath only results in our feeling even worse.

Take a moment to examine the following list and determine if negative, evaluative self-talk dominates *your* thoughts. Are you a…

Doubter: "I can't do this!"

Should-er: "I should be doing better."

Name caller: "I'm so stupid!"

Pessimist: "I will never get there."

Judge: "I am so fat!"

Comparison maker: "She is so much skinnier than I am."

Complainer: "This is so awful!"

How often do you entertain thoughts like the ones listed above? Is it any surprise that making comments like these to yourself is a major form of self-sabotage? Worse, if you engage in this unproductive criticism—filled with "shoulds" and "can'ts"—you're welcoming stress, anxiety, and other negative emotions into your life. And although this downward spiral can be difficult to escape, it's imperative to put the brakes on negative self-talk. If you don't, then you're likely to resort to food to self-soothe.

Being more mindful of your inner self-talk will allow you to shift the conversation from negative to more neutral or positive language. Even better, you can start to *soothe* yourself with positive self-talk (and simultaneously stop the trigger of emotional eating).

During the next week, pay close attention to the words you say to yourself. At the first hint of negative self-talk, use the following exercises to halt those unproductive thoughts in their tracks.

Soothing Strategy
Critical to Curious

The goal of this exercise is to learn to simply recognize when your inner voice is being downright mean and then get to the bottom of it.

- **Be mindful.** Don't let the inner criticism fly by without flagging it down and giving yourself a gentle nudge. You may even give it a name by saying, "Oh look, my Badgering Voice is back again." Or "Oh, my Miss Must-Be-Perfect voice is blathering on."

- **Be curious, not critical.** I always ask my clients inquisitively in counseling, "Where did that come from?" Ask yourself questions: "Is that my own voice talking or the echo of a critical parent? What triggered that thought? How does that thought make me feel?"

- **Is it true?** Now that you've gotten a wider perspective on the thought, ask yourself, "Is that a fact?" This step of the exercise may be difficult. Our thoughts are not often facts but opinions. Yet, we treat them like facts. Would a best friend agree with your thought? Probably not.

- **Distance yourself from the thought.** It can be helpful to step back from the thought and shake it loose a little by saying, "I'm having the thought that…" Notice how different this sounds: "I am so fat!" versus "I am having the thought that I am so fat." This kind of distance can cool down the intensity of the inner critic and remind you that a thought is just a thought.

Soothing Strategy
Use the Third Person

A recent study found that small shifts in your language can make a big difference in your self-talk (Kross et al. 2014). Instead of using first-person speech ("I") try using third-person language—that is, using your name—to distance yourself from the feeling. (You can even use the second-person "you.") It may feel a little strange at first. However, notice the shift in your emotions. Do they cool down when you refer to them from a distance?

Here's an example from a famous basketball player who used this technique. The player said during an interview, "One thing I didn't want to do was make an emotional decision. I wanted to do what's best for LeBron James and to do what makes LeBron James happy." Using one's own name versus using "I," a seemingly small shift in words, can be a helpful trick when introspectively thinking about something that is triggering hot emotions that lead to emotional eating.

No one can make you feel inferior without your consent.
—Eleanor Roosevelt

4. Mindful Tech: Caution!

Take a moment to answer these questions: Do you eat breakfast, lunch, or dinner with your phone? Do you check it at least once while you eat? Do you take your phone to the bathroom? Do your friends and family get annoyed with the amount of time you spend on your phone or computer? If so, you may be overly dependent on technology.

The irony of technology is that it makes it both easier and more difficult to connect with others. On one hand, it's a blessing, connecting you with former roommates and family across the continent, as well as allowing you to keep tabs on your network of friends and acquaintances. Geography and time zones are no longer a barrier, and the instantaneous nature of technology makes it affordable, quick, and easy to keep in touch with others.

However, technology can become a problem when you can no longer deal or even cope with the moment without it, or when you disconnect completely from your feelings for long periods of time. The point can't be hit home enough—you need your feelings to help inform your decisions, particularly food decisions.

In and of itself, these moments don't pose a problem; but a pattern of numbing yourself completely with food or technology will eventually prevent you from really dealing with your problems. Plus, there's a risk of the double-whammy: numbing out with technology *while* you eat for emotional reasons. We've all done it at one time or another—mindlessly munching as you sit at the computer, or eating your dinner as you chat on the phone or watch TV. As with everything, the occasional mindless meal isn't the issue; it's when eating and technology meld and become an ingrained behavioral habit.

Clients often "accidentally" leave their phones on during counseling. I've noticed that when their phones beep, alerting them of an e-mail, text message, or other notification, their train of thought stops and their attention is momentarily pulled to the phone. Although they may not look at their phone, their voice trails off; they're no longer in the moment telling their story. They are thinking, "I wonder who that is?" Some of my clients despise their phone, particularly those who are on call 24/7. It signals anxiety and the anticipation of being needed at all hours of the day and night. In other words, they know that their attention will be taken away from the present moment the minute the phone dings.

An interesting study on cell phones and students found that high-frequency cell phone users tended to have lower GPAs, higher anxiety, and lower satisfaction (unhappiness) with life relative to their peers who used the cell phone less often (Lepp, Barkley, and Karpinski 2014). In fact, another study found that even the small beeps and buzzes from our smartphones and tablets are not only disrupting our romantic relationships but hindering them as well (McDaniel and Coyne 2014). The survey asked more than one hundred women in cohabitating relationships how interruptive their smartphones and other devices were with their partners. Sixty-two percent of the women said technology interferes at least once a day if not more with their free time together.

Let's look at the technology aspect first. Where do *you* fall on the continuum? Is technology making your life easier, or is it taking it over? Consider the following:

- Start by observing how often you check your phone during the day.

- Ask yourself, "Am I looking at my phone to connect—or to disconnect?" If the answer is to disconnect from feelings, ask yourself, "What am I feeling? Bored? Tired? Frustrated?" Get in touch with your emotions. Can your phone or computer really provide you with what you need? Usually, the answer is no.

- If you're feeling negative emotions, remember to do your best to sit with those feelings, experience them, and feel them as they reach a crescendo and then begin to subside. Many times, when the feelings pass, you're less likely to rely on your technology as an emotional crutch.

If you find that your technology has more control over you than you'd like, try the following exercises.

Soothing Strategy
The Tech Emotional Makeover

- **Take a tech break.** When you catch yourself numbing out with technology, give yourself a time-out: 2 to 10 minutes without being connected. A few quiet moments to calm and soothe is a wonderful interruption, and after your time-out, make it your goal to reengage with others. Take a deep breath. Move. Talk. Be present.

- **Unplug completely.** As another experiment, go a few hours or a whole day without technology, and see how you feel when you don't have your phone, tablet, computer, or other device available to regulate your feelings. Be mindful of what happens when you take it away. Do you feel anxious? Bored? Sometimes this experiment helps people to realize how heavily they depend on their technology not just for connection but for managing their emotions.

- **Move it out of reach.** The next time you're out with other people, put your technology out of reach. Zip your phone into your purse, leave the laptop in your car, and so on. If you need to leave your phone on because you have children or a spouse or parent who may need to be in touch in case of an emergency, turn the phone to vibrate and place it on the table more than an arm's length away. If there's an emergency, you'll still be available, but you won't be as tempted to mindlessly check your phone, e-mail, or text messages.

Soothing Strategy
Silent Lunch

Phones don't make good dining companions. Technology can take you out of the moment, which is the opposite of mindful eating. Being fully present when you eat is difficult to do when your mind is buried in a newsfeed or scrolling through posts. You don't fully experience each bite, which leaves you at high risk for overeating and out-of-control emotional eating. This goes for eating at your desk, too. When it's time for lunch, walk away from your desk and go sit on a bench or in the break room.

The next time you're ready to eat, try these tech-free ideas to enjoy your food and dining companions more fully and mindfully:

- Strategically place your phone away from where you're sitting, either out of sight, in another room, or at least out of reach.

- When at work, move to another room to eat, or ask a friend to meet you out for lunch. If you *must* eat at your desk, swivel away from your computer screen and phone.

● Turn off the sound on your technology. Even a beep can distract you from focusing on what you are eating and who you are with.

The more ways we have to connect, the more many of us seem desperate to unplug. —Pico Iyer

5. Mindfully Plug In

In the previous chapter, we looked at some of the ways technology can inhibit your ability to be mindful and how it can contribute to emotional eating. But when used thoughtfully and judiciously, it *can* enhance your life.

In this section are ten ways to use technology to promote soothing. Each idea is coupled with the emotions you may be experiencing at the time. By using the technology to soothe rather than "numb out," you can reengage with the world much more mindfully than if you use food to hide your emotions. Plus, most of us take our phones with us everywhere we go—make this a great opportunity to use the phone appropriately and enjoy another positive benefit from it.

Another perk? Technology provides amazing opportunities to track your energy level, sleep patterns, mood, foods eaten, exercise, blood pressure, and so on. All of these biological metrics and factors can help you keep closer track of your mood and hand you very clear data on exactly what triggers emotional eating. Clients who use their phones to document their mood in the moment rather than hours later in a journal (when they can lose or forget information) have a better handle on their emotions. For example, if you have the urge to munch when you are not truly hungry, whipping out your phone and entering data on what you're feeling right at that very moment can give you valuable information on what is driving that urge to eat. It's easier to decode right then and there.

A study in the *Annals of Internal Medicine* found that overweight participants who were committed to using a health app to track eating, calories, and other data lost more weight than those who didn't use such a system (Laing et al. 2014). My own clients have sang the praises of their technology in helping them manage their mood and steer clear of emotional eating. Chances are, your smartphone is almost always just an arm's reach away. Plus, the ease of recording one's mood with an app has replaced the sometimes cumbersome task of carrying a paper journal.

The downside is that not everyone has fancy technology to keep his or her mind occupied. If you don't, that's okay. You can still adapt the suggestions to a low-tech version by using a small notebook or pad of paper. Always remember: It's important to balance this technique with others, as technology can also yank you out of the moment. We're shooting for a healthy balance.

Soothing Strategy
Ten Ways to Use Tech to Track

First, identify what you are feeling. Then, choose one of the following options:

- *When you're bored or anxious:* Play a game or crossword puzzle online—or the low-tech way, on paper.

- *When you need connection:* Check your e-mail. Low-tech method: phone a friend.

- *When you're feeling overwhelmed or upset:* Journal your feelings and thoughts.

- *When you want to boost your self-esteem:* Post a positive message to a friend; doing something nice for others will make you feel better, too!

- *When you're feeling lonely:* Check social media to see what your friends are doing. Low-tech way: check in with a neighbor or work colleague.

- *When you can't sleep, feel upset, or can't turn off your mind:* Choose a "relaxation" or "meditation" app. Low-tech way: read about the five types of meditation discussed in part II of this book.

- *When you're feeling anxious, stressed, or bored:* Play music that is soothing or calming; some music can be stimulating, so be sure to find something that relaxes you.

- *When you're irritated, angry, or bored:* Check the weather to interrupt your negative feelings.

- *When you're wallowing:* Check the news. It's a good reminder that there are more important and even worse things happening in the world. This is not to downplay what you're going through, but it can help to give perspective.

own.** First, sit down. Bring the food up to your mouth
d of leaning in or forward to meet your food. Pay
attention to how your body moves and bridges the gap
en your food and mouth. Sometimes your body auto-
ally slumps as you eat, so be aware of your posture.
nue to maintain this erect posture during meals. Notice
he positioning of your body actually shifts your mood
vay of eating.

ly chew.** As you eat the food, take your time. Chew
y. Try to chew each bite of food at least twenty to thirty
. In addition to slowing you down, chewing thoroughly
id with digestion. Another way to slow your eating is
t your eating utensil down in between bites. Think of it
vay: pausing between bites allows you to fully focus on
conversation, since you're not talking with an awkward
hful of food!

se.** Use your senses. Look at your food. Notice the
s, presentation, and arrangement on your plate. Take
to appreciate what you are about to eat. Also take a
ent to enjoy the smell of your food before eating. When
restaurant, notice how prettily your food is plated.

or.** Appreciate the taste, smell, and texture of your food.
t rush for the next bite, either. Remember that it takes
body approximately twenty minutes to recognize that

- *When you're bored:* Google a topic you've been curious
  about. Low-tech alternative: flip through a magazine
  and find an article you might not normally read.

Technology is a useful servant but a dangerous master.
—**Christian Lous Lange**

6. Consume Mindfully

Have you ever been sitting on the couch munching on chips when you got to the bottom of the bag and thought, "How did I eat so much?!" You never intended to empty the bag in one sitting! You suddenly go from feeling relaxed to distressed and guilty. One of the best antidotes to the bad feelings from mindless overeating is mind*ful* eating.

Mindful eaters are simply calmer around food. Since we know that food anxiety often leads to emotional eating, having mindful eating skills in your pocket helps you be more composed and in charge of your eating habits. So when you're faced with stress, you can handle food wisely with confidence.

Mindful eaters tend to use food less often than others to manage their emotions. They also tend to have healthier eating habits and smaller portion sizes. So building up this skill is important.

Mindless eating leads to a lot of accidental stress, guilt, and all-around awful feelings. No one means to mindlessly eat. It's really just a symptom of being disconnected from your body. Eating while driving, having a conversation, watching TV, using technology, and even during negative self-talk are all too common occurrences for many people. But mealtime doesn't have to be laden with anxiety and guilt. The key? Always being plugged in and tuned in to your body—particularly when you eat.

The benefits of mindful eating are bo[th] numerous. In fact, one study found that those were able to shift their eating behaviors, alte[r] reduce psychological distress (Dalen et al. 2[0] study found that in addition to the aforem[entioned] mindfulness at mealtime could positively af[fect] index (Godfrey, Gallo, and Afari 2015). Tha[t] ranks foods on a scale of 1 to 100 based on [their] blood sugar levels. And for those who bing[e] can reduce the frequency of bingeing episode[s] of anxiety (Godfrey, Gallo, and Afari 2015)[.] powerful benefits to receive, all from payin[g] you eat, right?

Soothing Strate[gy]
Five S's of Mindful E[ating]

Follow these steps to increase mindfulness your food. For best results, practice mindful *not* feeling stressed. That way, when you e[at] percent connected to your body. Also, sch[edule] time to eat so that you can take advantage [of] mentioned in the technology chapters, you'll electronics to allow yourself to really enjoy th[e] without distraction.

you're full. Being mindful and taking your time will allow you to become aware of satiety levels, and the slower you eat, the greater your odds for noticing when you're full—before you've eaten too much. Ultimately, this will result in eating less at each meal.

Smile. Intentionally smiling helps you take a pause between bites. In that gap, consider whether you are satisfied or want to keep eating.

When practiced to its fullest, mindful eating turns a simple meal into a spiritual experience, giving us a deep appreciation of all that went into the meal's creation as well as a deep understanding of the relationship between the food on our table, our own health, and our planet's health. —Thich Nhat Hanh

7. Biofeedback

Before you think that biofeedback therapy is too technical or too much mumbo jumbo to learn, trust me, it's fairly simple. We often use food as a "pseudo biofeedback machine," trying to change our physiology—our stress level—with a hunk of chocolate or an order of french fries. Think about that for a minute. It is fascinating that we expect what we eat to change our physiology, right? Biofeedback therapy is training yourself to alter physiological processes such as blood pressure, heart rate, and muscle tension. All that means is you're using your body's own biological data to help you understand how you feel.

This isn't so foreign. If you've ever taken your temperature to find out if you have a fever, or stepped on a scale to know how much you weigh, or used a tape measure to determine your waist circumference, you've already used elements of biofeedback. These tools tell you what you need to know about your own body so you can monitor it more effectively—the number on the scale, for instance, reveals if you need to eat less or more, or whether you're just right; the high temperature of the fever indicates the need for some action, like getting some rest, putting a cool washcloth on your head, and drinking fluids. The beauty of biofeedback is that it gives you actual data that you can track.

Teaching people biofeedback has been helpful in reducing emotional eating. One study showed that after having eight sessions of biofeedback, women with a body mass index of more than thirty-five learned better self-efficacy (felt more empowered to make changes) and were better able to control their stress levels, eating behaviors, and relaxation (Teufel et al. 2013).

Those who have practiced biofeedback have found relief from numerous conditions, such as headaches, high blood pressure, stress, insomnia, pain, depression, and more. By using biofeedback, you can learn to relax and unwind your mind, allowing you to de-stress in a healthy way. Indeed, the mind-body connection that is inherent to biofeedback gives you yet another avenue for dealing with uncomfortable feelings—without turning to food. As an added benefit, you may be able to put an end to other nagging health conditions at the same time!

Soothing Strategy
Download an App

In the past, biofeedback machines were complicated and very expensive—hundreds even thousands of dollars. You often had to visit the doctor's office for weekly therapy. Now, if you have a smartphone, you can have your very own biofeedback machine. In the app store, look for two kinds of apps: one that will change the pace of your breathing (you match the rate of the app with your breath), and one that measures your heart rate. Here are some popular apps:

- **BellyBio Interactive Breathing:** This app monitors breathing and plays sounds like ocean waves to help you relax. It's great for anxiety and stress (iPhone only).

- **iBiofeedback:** This heart rate monitor has you put your finger over the camera to assess your heart rate. It's simple and the app is free.

- **BioZen:** If you enjoy biofeedback and are interested in using it often, some apps require you to buy an attachment (for example, one clamps on the ear or on your finger) that you sync to your body to gather your biological data (such as brain waves, galvanic skin response, heart rate, respiratory rate, temperature, and more). BioZen is one such app.

If you don't have a smartphone, you can still learn to get to know your body's cues. With practice, you can learn some of the information the old-fashioned way: by simply placing your fingers on your wrist and taking your pulse.

Soothing Strategy
Master Your Mind

To calm down your body and mind, find a quiet place where you can concentrate for 10 to 15 minutes. Close your eyes and visualize a pleasant scene. Imagine any location that makes you feel more serene. Here are just a few ideas:

- **For beach lovers:** Picture a white-sand beach, with waves gently rolling to the shore. The sun is shining, and the sky is clear blue without a single cloud in sight. Maybe you are floating in the ocean gazing upward.

- **For forest lovers:** You're walking through the woods and observing the tall trees, green leaves, and cool, soft ground beneath your feet. You can hear the birds chirping as the sun peeks through the foliage to warm your skin.

- **For hikers and climbers:** You're sitting on a rock after a day of hiking and climbing. You look out at the valley below you, a colorful expanse of rooftops, green grass, and trees. A cool breeze moves through the air, and you can feel the sun on your skin.

Be sure to choose a visual that matches your preferences and personality. If there's another scene that inspires you, use that for your visualization!

Soothing Strategy
More Ways to Lower Your Heart Rate

Here are a few more ways you can lower your heart rate. As you experiment with biofeedback, take note of your stress level and emotions. Over time, biofeedback can help you feel more relaxed and less tempted to eat for emotional reasons.

- **Go auditory.** Some people gain the most benefit by repeating words and phrases as a way to focus their thoughts and dip into a calm state of being. The repetition puts yourself in a more suggestible state that ultimately allows you to relax. Come up with your own words, or chose from this list: *Warmth... My hands are warm and heavy... Heat... Light... Love warms my heart...*

- **Follow your breath.** Paying attention to your breathing is another excellent way to relax your body and mind. Simply close your eyes and notice where you're breathing from: Is it the chest or the belly? Are you breathing deeply, or is your breath shallow? Are you breathing quickly or slowly? Also note how your nostrils flare on the exhalation and contract on the inhalation. Keep bringing your awareness back to these aspects of your breath. (You'll find more breathing techniques in Part III: Mindful Breathing.)

- **Warm your hands.** Another exercise that can relax tense parts of your body is *external* hand warming. The technique is simple: Rub your hands together, and continue to rub until you feel the heat. Then place your hand on a body part that needs soothing. For instance, placing your palms over your eyes is calming. And the calmer you feel, the more mindful you'll be, and subsequently less prone to emotional eating.

To understand any living thing, you must, so to say, creep within and feel the beating of its heart. —W. Macneile Dixon

8. Distraction

Does the following scenario sound familiar? As you spoon out chunks of chocolate brownie ice cream directly from the container, you say to yourself, "This is so good, but I *have* to stop. Right now. But just one more bite. Oh, there is another brownie bite. So good. Now I'll stop. Now. Wait, just one more bite. Now really I'll stop. Agh!" You just can't seem to tear yourself away from the throes of emotional eating even when you give yourself a direct command to quit eating right now!

Then your phone rings. It's your close friend, and you become immersed in a conversation, completely forgetting about the ice cream your mind insisted it had to have a few minutes ago. You put the rest of the carton away without even the slightest hesitation. Later, you think to yourself, "Wow, I felt like I couldn't tear myself away from the ice cream, but then I just completely forgot about it. I didn't even give it a second thought." Welcome to the amazing power of distraction.

Distraction can play both a positive and negative role in your life. Being distracted, like texting while you are driving, is not only difficult; it can be fatal. Distracting yourself while you eat—such as typing on the computer while eating pretzels, or reading a novel while you eat dinner—isn't recommended, since you can't be mindful of the process or when you become full. In fact, being distracted while eating can lead to overeating. For example, watching TV while eating is a huge trigger for overeating (Braude and Stevenson 2014). One study in the *Journal of the American Medical Association* found that people who watched an action movie snacked more than those who didn't snack in front of the TV, even with the sound off (Chapman et al. 2014).

What's more, eating while distracted leads to enjoying food less. A study in the journal *Psychological Science* found that when people eat and drink while distracted, they require greater concentrations of sweetness, sourness, or saltiness to feel satisfied (van der Wal and van Dillen 2013). In other words, you may be more likely to notice a subtle spice when you're concentrating on each bite. However, food can taste bland if you eat while your attention is divided.

That said, you can use a diversion or distraction to your benefit when it is *purposeful* and *intentional*. Distraction can shake loose thoughts of eating and put an end to the loop of food chatter that makes you mindlessly munch. It takes your attention and focus off strong emotions and unproductive thoughts. By giving yourself something else to do or focus on, you give yourself time for the thought about food or the emotion driving you to eat to cool down and dissipate, making it easier to cope. It's like a thunderstorm reducing to a light rain. Distraction is not escaping your feelings (as it is when you do anything that smothers or erases feelings, like drinking or binge eating); it's a form of coping.

In a study presented at the Obesity Society (2014) conference, researchers tested the effects of three thirty-second distraction techniques that reduce cravings for favorite foods. The first, tapping one's own forehead and ear with the index finger; the second, tapping one's toe on the floor; and the third, staring at a blank wall, all worked to significantly reduce cravings. In this study, researchers found that the forehead tapping worked the best. Although it is unclear why this works, one could hypothesize that this action is so far out of the range of things you would normally do that it would likely take some effort and concentration—enough to distract you from your current thoughts.

Again, I've found that the benefit from distraction comes when it's *intentional* distraction—when you choose where to place your attention and then give your all to that activity. For example, if you're munching on potato chips, decide to send an e-mail as a way to stop eating. This is in contrast to the distraction that divides your attention between two tasks, as in driving while texting, which forces you to switch back and forth between each task. A good intentional distraction is one that requires you to stop eating, stop looking for food, and stop thinking about food in order to perform the task. It should divert *all* your attention from eating. There are many ways we can distract ourselves. You can color, watch a movie, play a game on your phone, clean, do a puzzle, organize, e-mail a friend. Virtually any activity is fodder for a distraction.

Soothing Strategy
5-5-5-5-5 Exercise

When you feel the urge to emotionally eat, it's important to move and act in a new way. This technique is one I created, and it's a favorite of mine. Remember that to use distraction effectively, give the activity 100 percent of your attention for a specific amount of time—enough to allow the stress or craving feelings you are experiencing to dampen down.

Get out a piece of paper and write down:

- **5 people** (friend, parent, etc.) you can call when you feel down or upset, or need to vent

- **5 ways you relax** (take a hot shower, shut your eyes, put your feet up, etc.)

- **5 places you go to calm down** (your bed, a quiet room where people can't bother you, outdoors, etc.)

- **5 things you can say to yourself** ("I can do this!" "This too will pass," etc.)

- **5 activities to distract yourself** (start a puzzle, watch a movie, run an errand, etc.)

Hang this list in an easy-to-see location, like on your refrigerator or cupboard, and look at it when you need a reminder to create a diversion. Then do the diversion for at least 5 minutes!

Soothing Strategy
Anti-Dwell Techniques Refocus and Reframe

A distraction doesn't have to include physical activities like running, crafting, or cleaning. A distraction can simply be another thought. When dwelling on food or other feelings, try to break loose by diving into a new thought.

You know how unproductive it is to tell yourself, "Stop thinking about the leftover pizza in the refrigerator." That never works! A study out of Ohio State indicates that it's more helpful to have specific things to think about. Trying to suppress or turn off your thinking sometimes leads to a rebound effect of craving a food even more. People in the study who were instructed on how to distract themselves, versus those who just dwelled on their thoughts, had a decrease in cortisol, the stress hormone (Zoccola et al. 2014). And when you're less stressed, it's easier to fight off cravings.

Here's how to do it. First, commit to 5 minutes of what I call Refocus and Reframe. Close your eyes. Then pick one:

- Fantasize about your future career.

- Imagine where you would like to go on vacation.

- Visualize floating on waves in the ocean.

- Imagine yourself walking down the aisle of a furniture store.

- Think about someone you'd like to kiss right now.

- Imagine doing something wild and out of character for you.

- Remember the funniest incident you can think of.

Write down a few prompts of your own. Revisit these scenarios anytime the urge to comfort eat pulls you toward the pantry.

Distracted by all sorts of distractions, it wanders around aimlessly in the ten directions. —Sri Guru Granth Sahib

9. Grounding Techniques

Have you ever been so trapped in your thoughts and feelings that you lost big chunks of time without even really realizing it? Or you were dwelling on something so fully that you turned down the wrong hallway and then said, "Wait, where was I going?"

Maybe you are feeling so depressed that you just want to stay in bed. Or you are so angry or anxious or stressed that it's having an impact on your work and other duties—you can't seem to concentrate on tasks or follow simple directions. That's when you know your emotions have taken over and are in control.

Grounding techniques are a powerful way to support yourself through heavy emotional times. They help to bring you back to the present moment, preventing you from being swept away by your feelings and resorting to mindlessly eating comfort foods. They work to physically and mentally "ground" you to the earth and this moment; they can be a touchstone that lets you know you are okay, that you can get through this, that you will come out the other side in tact—without hitting the fridge or the office vending machine.

Grounding techniques work by helping you to focus on what is happening outside yourself rather than what is going on inside. The word "grounding" may remind you of electricity. We need to ground an electric line before we work with it and to make it safe. Think of your feelings like this electric line, needing to be grounded to make them more welcoming and user friendly.

Soothing Strategy
How to Ground Yourself

Grounding techniques often use the five senses (sound, touch, smell, taste, and sight). They aim to immediately connect you to the here and now, to bring you back to the moment rather than dwell on your feelings. All the grounding techniques produce sensations that are difficult to ignore, thereby directly and instantaneously connecting you with the present moment.

Grounding Your Body

To anchor your physical body to the present, choose one of these to try:

- Listen to loud music.

- Hold on to a piece of ice.

- Bite into a lemon or grapefruit.

- Place your hands under cool or hot water, or place a wet washcloth on a part of your body.

- Stop in place. Push your heels against the floor as if digging into it. Literally ground yourself.

- Carry a soothing object in your hand or pocket. A smooth stone, for example, is something that you can rub or clutch when feeling upset.

- Sit down, grab the arms of a chair, and grip them tightly. Release.

- Shake your hands, then clench, and let go. Repeat.

Grounding Your Mind

These tips are designed to help you stop or disengage from your thoughts. By focusing strategically on something else, you can lessen your distress.

- Read a passage from a book backward out loud starting at the end and going forward. This takes much more concentration than reading forward.

- Choose a "getaway" image. For example, imagine jumping into a fancy, fast sports car and driving away from the source of your stress. Or imagine tying your feelings to a hot air balloon and watching them float into the air.

- Stewing about the past? Repeat a mantra that brings you back to the moment, such as, "This moment is okay. I can't control the past or the future, but now I am okay."

- Do you feel like you are having a meltdown like a two-year-old? Maybe you feel like you have regressed by curling into a ball, stomping your feet, or pouting. Identify the age you're acting, then start to work your way up to your current age. Tell yourself, "Now I am moving into age three" and continue to count slowly up. Take on the posture of each age.

- Recite a list. Choose a group of things you can list, like all the U.S. states. Think of as many as you can, along with their capitals. Or try naming cities that start with P, things that are the color red, and so on.

- Repeat song lyrics.

- Flip through the pictures on your phone.

Grounding to the Earth

Sometimes it takes connecting directly with the earth to help overcome overwhelming, distracting emotions. Here are a few suggestions to do this:

- Take your shoes off and feel your feet against the ground. Better yet, go for a walk outside on grass or at the beach, if possible.

- Dig your hands into some dirt. This is a good time to do some gardening!

- Sit on the floor, place your hands on the ground, and notice your connection to the earth.

- Walk up to a tree and rub your hands over the bark, noticing its textures.

Let's not forget that the little emotions are the great captains of our lives and we obey them without realizing it. —Vincent van Gogh

Meditation

"Meditation practice isn't about trying to throw ourselves away and become something better, it's about befriending who we are." This quote from Buddhist teacher and author Ani Pema Chödrön gives us a great clue as to what meditation is all about. Underneath all the mind chatter and mental distortions is a place of peace and quiet, and meditation is the tool to take you there!

In this chapter, I provide you with five different types of meditation. I encourage you to try all five and see which you connect with most. Once you do find a meditation technique you like, stick with it for a while, practicing regularly, to reap the most benefits. There is an old and wise saying: "To find water, dig deep."

10. Focus Meditation

Picture yourself at the dinner table eating chicken and vegetables, when all of a sudden your mind wanders back to some distant memory, perhaps you eating in the kitchen of your childhood. You're transported there, picturing your parents and siblings, hearing their conversations, being amused by the jokes or enthralled by the smells... No wonder you ate way more than you intended—you were lost in thoughts far, far away!

Many of us can be easily transported back in time through hearing a favorite song on the radio, smelling some familiar odor, or daydreaming about a better time or a sad loss we once experienced. But memories aren't the only things that pull our focus away; everyday items like the Internet, television, people we're surrounded by, and so on can destroy our attention span too. My clients often say, "It was like I suddenly woke up and realized that I had eaten the entire bag of cheese puffs!"

Maybe you let your mind wander at work, during a boring task, or while driving mindlessly on your commute home. A recent study of more than 2,000 adults found that 47 percent of the time their mind wasn't on the task at hand (Killingsworth and Gilbert 2010). Worse, people reported that they were less happy when their mind wandered. The study suggests it may be helpful (on many levels) to learn to keep the mind from wandering off and learn to focus more fully in the present.

The good news is that with practice, you can train yourself to place your attention where you want it to be. Focused-attention meditation can help you accomplish this. What's more, it may also improve your memory. In a study at the University of California, Santa Barbara, forty-eight undergrad students took either a mindfulness or nutrition course (Mrazek et al. 2013). The mindfulness course focused on meditation. Afterward, all the students took the GRE, the standardized test for grad school admittance. Students who took the mindfulness course outperformed students who took the nutrition course, and their working memory and focus improved.

Focus meditation can be a powerful tool in your arsenal of tricks against mindlessly munching on foods while your thoughts are somewhere else. Use it to learn to stay focused when eating or doing any important task. It may seem difficult at first, but the more you practice, the easier focused meditation becomes. Go ahead—you too can meditate!

Soothing Strategy
Single-Minded Meditation

Being trapped in your head or by your thoughts pulls you out of the present moment. Try this focused meditation to stay in the present moment and turn off or down your internal dialogue.

Sit in a comfortable upright position, either on the floor or in a chair. Make sure your torso is right over your hips and that your head, neck, and spine are in one line. Choose one thing to focus on. It can be something directly in front of you like a picture, a chair, or a spot on the wall. Focus for 3 minutes (set the timer on your watch or phone). Using all of your senses, describe the object in as much detail as possible. What does it smell like? Look like? Sound like?

If your mind starts to analyze what you're doing, wanders from the object, or gets bored, notice this thought and gently bring your mind back to the moment to continue describing the object. It's very common for your mind to wander, but as you practice this meditation, your ability to stay focused will increase. Just as you build strength in your muscles when you exercise, you will build strength in your capacity to focus and be present the more you practice. Start with a few minutes and work up to 8 to 10 minutes over time and as your schedule allows.

Soothing Strategy
Candle Gazing

In yoga, the practice of gazing at a candle is called *tratak* or "forehead wash." It is a very powerful method for increasing concentration, focus, and memory. Candle gazing also clears the tear ducts and helps some eye problems. *Note:* If you have cataracts or are epileptic do *not* practice with flame. Instead, use a stationary object such as a pinpoint on paper, a flower, a leaf, or something similar.

First, gather a chair, candle, match, or lighter, and a small plate. Start by sitting on the floor with the chair 3 to 4 feet in front of you. Place the candle on a plate or some other device to catch the melting wax and protect the chair. Light the candle and make sure that the flame is approximately at eye level.

As you sit in a comfortable position, begin to take slow deep breaths. Continue to breathe slowly, gazing at the flame. You want to look at the base of the flame. Keep your eyes open and avoid blinking as much as possible until you feel your eyes start to tear, approximately 3 to 4 minutes, and then close your eyes.

Now look for the image of the flame in your mind's eye. It may start to move around, and you will want to work to bring it back to the center of your mind. When you can no longer see the image inside, open your eyes and repeat the whole process again up to three or four times.

Soothing Strategy
Balance on One Leg

A quick way to get highly focused is to challenge your balance.

Begin by standing 6 to 8 inches from a wall, facing it. Place your fingertips about mid-chest level on the wall, bend your right knee, and lift your right foot off the ground so that you are balanced on your left foot. Find a spot on the wall to stare at. Experiment with taking your fingers off the wall. Stay here for 1 to 2 minutes, if possible, and then switch to the other side. Not only will you find this a great exercise for focusing, it will improve your balance too!

Concentrate all your thoughts upon the work at hand. The sun's rays do not burn until brought to a focus. —Alexander Graham Bell

11. Vipassana Meditation

Also known as "Insight Meditation," Vipassana is designed to do just what its translation suggests: provide ultimate insight into how your mind works and, through this process, reveal the true nature of your reality. Vipassana is said to be the same method of meditation that Buddha used and taught some 2,500 years ago. And while Vipassana is definitely associated with Buddhism, the meditation itself is nondenominational and practiced by many different people all over the world.

The practice of Vipassana, like most meditation practices, helps you learn to become present and mindful of what is happening in the moment. Most of us experience lots of internal suffering because we replay thoughts and feelings about something that happened in the past or fantasize about something that may or may not occur in the future. In this way, Vipassana is an ideal antidote to emotional eating. When you're eating because of buried feelings, you're not present in the moment but rather consciously or subconsciously numbing your emotions with food. By learning to be present more often, you will be less likely to let emotions govern your choices; instead you will learn to identify them as they crop up.

Through regular Vipassana practice, you may find that many desires and troubling thoughts simply fade away; at the same time, you may develop more compassion for yourself and others. Not surprising, modern research is showing that Vipassana is extremely helpful for improving your overall well-being—including reducing depression, anxiety, and stress—and the functioning of your brain (Chiesa 2010; Szekeres and Wertheim 2014).

If you've struggled with food cravings, you know how much suffering food issues can cause. Carmen, one of my clients, didn't want food cravings to get the best of her anymore. Slowing down and turning to Vipassana was the exact tool she needed to obtain a steadfast refusal to give in to the thought "I want chocolate!" The technique reminded her that cravings are transient. They come, they go. They aren't permanent, and not responding to them immediately gives them time to transform and change. They often go away when you give them an opportunity to take leave.

Carmen said, "I used to have food cravings, and I thought that I had to answer them immediately. Once I started to become less attached to my thoughts through Vipassana, I could easily examine a craving in detail by talking it through in my head. I'd say, 'Okay, Carmen, you're having a craving for ice cream right now. Why is that? Well, let's think... Today was a tough day at work and there's that big review tomorrow at the office. Plus, Mark is away on business and I always find the evenings a little lackluster and lonely when he's not here. I think I'm a little anxious and bored—a bad combination that brings on my need to eat something creamy and comforting... I'll read this new novel until it passes and that should help."

Soothing Strategy
Rise and Release

When you feel the urge to escape your feelings with food, try this:

Begin by sitting on the floor or in a chair. Bring your torso right over your hips and be sure to sit up straight with your head, neck, and spine in one line.

Close your eyes and bring your awareness to your breath, not changing it or altering it in any way. Imagine pressing the "mute" button on your TV. You are just silently watching and observing what is happening. Notice how your belly and chest move in and out with your breath. To become even more aware of your experience in the moment, mentally say the word "rising" as your belly expands on the inhalation, and say the word "releasing" as you exhale.

Most likely your focus will begin to wander. You might have visual images or memories or feel something in your body, or an emotion will come to the surface; you might hear something outside, or have the urge to talk to yourself. When this occurs, simply name what it is and then return your awareness back to the rising and falling of your breath. For example, if you are picturing something, name it—"visualizing"—and return to the present. If it is an emotion, simply name it—"anger" or "grief" or "anxiety"—and when you hear something, name what you hear: "birds," "neighbors," "kids playing," "traffic," and so on.

Start by practicing for 5 minutes, working up to 30 minutes or more as your schedule allows.

Soothing Strategy
Giving Your Cravings the Silent Treatment

When you have a craving, try *really* listening to it while doing a moment-to-moment examination of the body. Or if there is a time of day when you regularly find yourself eating for emotional reasons, experiment with a little preplanning: Have a meditation session just a few minutes prior to when that craving might occur. When cravings do occur, simply notice them and name them as cravings. Allow them, but distance yourself from them as if you were a scientist studying and watching them. Use calmness and focused attention. Here is how:

First, sit in a comfortable, relaxed, but alert way. Breathe naturally, without changing your breath. You can focus on the breath by silently saying to yourself "in" or "rising" with the inhalation and "out" or "falling" with the exhalation.

Start at the top of your head and work slowly down your body. Notice where the craving is taking place. Is it in your head? Is it giving you a headache or distracting you? Are you experiencing the craving in your mouth? Maybe you notice that you salivate as you start to think about the craving. Where is the pain or struggle coming from in your body?

Don't fight it. Just listen and identify all the places where the craving is coming from in your body. Remember that the goal isn't to squash cravings but to master control over them.

Continue to sit. Pay attention to any thoughts that go through your mind like, "Oh, this is agony. I can't stand it!" or "I feel like I am fighting myself."

When you are ready, open your eyes.

Half an hour's meditation each day is essential, except when you are busy. Then a full hour is needed. —Saint Francis de Sales

12. Mala Bead Meditation

You probably have seen people using or wearing mala beads—sometimes referred to as "prayer beads" or "worry beads"—around their wrists or necks. Essentially, they are a string of beads, usually 108 (the number 108 has various spiritual connotations), that are used as a focal point in meditation. There is one large head bead, known as the *meru* or the *guru*, in the string. Mala beads create a tactile focal point during meditation, as each bead is typically moved through the finger and thumb as described below. They allow you to focus on your meditation without worrying about how many times you should repeat your mantra.

Dating back to at least the tenth century, mala beads are made from a variety of different materials such as marble, gemstones, wood, or bone, and each material is said to have its own energy. They are often quite beautiful. A popular wood for mala beads is sandalwood, which is fragrant and said to encourage tranquility and a positive frame of mind. Beads made from clear crystals or mother of pearl are said to clear away obstacles like illness, calamities, and bad luck.

A study from Cambridge, England, found that doing something with your hands, such as fiddling with worry beads, may help alleviate trauma and stress (Holmes, Brewin, and Hennessy 2004). In this study, participants watched graphic footage of car accidents and then used various ways of keeping their hands busy, including striking a similar repetitive pattern on a keyboard, to feel better. Those who did verbal exercises like counting out loud had no relief, giving rise to the notion that working beads through your hands, fidgeting with objects, or squeezing stress balls can help. In fact, we have seen evidence of this kind of helpful action across the ages. While it sounds pretty gruesome, during the French Revolution, a group of people who watched the beheadings known as the *tricoteurs* knitted away as they watched hundreds of people lose their heads to the guillotine. Some suggest that their numb response may in part have been linked to the knitting.

Interestingly, more than two-thirds of the world's population use worry beads or prayer beads as part of their spiritual or meditative practices. But you don't need to belong to any religious or spiritual group to use them. Through practice, they will give a sense of grounding, focus, and peace of mind. Mala beads can be particularly beneficial if you are fidgety, very busy, eat quickly, or travel a lot, because you can take them with you wherever you go. And the more you practice with them, the quicker you will benefit from them, wherever you are.

Mala beads can be purchased on the Internet through a wide variety of websites. You can also find instructions on how to make your own if you are so inclined, or use any beaded bracelet.

Soothing Strategy
Meditating with Beads

To practice with mala beads, sit in a comfortable upright position on the floor or in a chair. Place the mala beads in your right hand and over either the ring finger or middle finger. Use your thumb to move from one bead to the next. The index finger is not used, as it represents the ego.

As you begin to touch each bead, simply count the beads, taking a slow breath between each. When you get to the head bead, turn back in the opposite direction until you touch the head bead again. Instead of counting, other options include repeating a prayer or mantra each time you touch a new bead. (See chapter 13, Mantra Meditation, for more information about mantras.)

Another great way to use mala beads is at the beginning or end of each day. When you go to sleep at night or wake up in the morning, hold the beads in your hand and notice the texture, weight, temperature, and color of the beads. Then think of what you are grateful for in your life, or set a positive intention for yourself, such as "I take care of my body" or "I eat healthy food that nourishes me."

The next time you are tempted to eat for emotional reasons, consider practicing a mala bead meditation instead. The practice will bring you right into the present moment, clear your mind, and balance your emotions.

Life is a train of moods like a string of beads; and as we pass through them they prove to be many colored lenses, which paint the world their own hue, and each shows us only what lies in its own focus. —Ralph Waldo Emerson

13. Mantra Meditation

Mantras are words, sounds, or phrases that help you focus your mind. In the process of repeating the mantra over and over, you can turn down your mind's inner noise and chaos. Mantras can deliver you to a more meditative state. They're intended to help you put down your to-do list and all the things clogging up your mind and focus your attention inward. Interestingly, the word "mantra" itself means "to protect," as in "to protect the mind."

Mantras have been used by many different traditions throughout time including Hinduism, Buddhism, Jainism, Sikhism, and Yoga, just to name a few. Similarly, chants, hymns, and prayers, which show up in almost every spiritual or religious tradition, can produce comparable effects and benefits.

There are many old and classical mantras that have withstood the test of time and are worth trying for their purported ability to produce a certain consciousness. But mantras can also be made up by any individual for any purpose. Self-chosen, affirming words can be like turning on the air conditioning in your brain—cooling off hot embers that fuel the fire of anger, loneliness, boredom, or frustration.

Research on mantras has found that they can actually change the blood flow in the part of your brain that controls motor and sensory functioning and memory. Chanting "om" has been shown to deactivate the brain structure's limbic system and the amygdala, which helps people manage emotion. In this study, subjects said either "om" or "sssss." Making the "sssss" sound didn't produce the same brain results (Kalyani et al. 2011).

For my client Katie, a biology major who struggles daily with stress eating due to a campus job and afternoon labs, mantras and chanting helped give her mind something else to do. It points her thoughts in a different direction and spreads a sense of inner calm by clearing out her daily worries. My clients use mantras, and so do I. If you took a peek into my house, you would see mantras stuck on mirrors, doors, and walls. Inspirational sayings help keep you positive!

What's more, studies show that chanting meditation improves the memory and cognitive brain function of people with memory-related problems (Newberg et al. 2010). The changes in the brain due to chanting meditation seem to be able to deactivate areas in the brain such as the left lobe—responsible for logic and analysis—which help to quiet it, creating the calming experience Katie has (Khalsa et al. 2009).

Soothing Strategy
Meditating with a Mantra

To practice mantra meditation, sit in a comfortable upright position on the floor or in a chair. Make sure your head, neck, and spine are in one line. Let your eyes close, and begin to repeat your chosen mantra over and over again. Start with 5 minutes and work up to 20 minutes over time, if you like.

Below are some traditional mantras as well as some that my clients have created for themselves that have proven effective. You can also use your own word or phrase that has meaning for you. Be sure to make it a positive word or statement. Feel free to experiment with them all and see which you like best. When you do find one you particularly like, stick with it for a while, as repeated practice will produce the best results. Mantras can be said silently to yourself or spoken out loud.

Traditional Mantras

- **"Om" or "Aum":** This is one of the oldest and simplest mantras. It's believed to be the sound of creation. All other sounds are said to come from "Aum." "Aum" is repeated over and over and over again.

- **"So hum":** This phrase means "I am that," which refers to spirit. "So" is said as you inhale and "hum" as you exhale.

- **"Om mani padme hum":** This is a classical mantra that can be found in many different cultures and spiritual practices. It literally means "jewel in the lotus" and alludes to the fact that we all have divinity within ourselves.

- **"Sa," "ta," "na," and "ma":** In the study on cognition mentioned above, participants chanted mantra meditations while touching their thumbs to their other fingers one at a time, saying "sa," "ta," "na," and "ma" respectively for each finger. They practiced the chanting meditation for twelve minutes: 2 minutes of chanting aloud, 2 minutes whispering the sounds, 4 minutes saying them silently, 2 minutes whispering again, and ending with 2 minutes of aloud chanting. Of course, you needn't follow such a protocol to give chanting meditation a try.

Healthy Eating Mantras

Throughout the years, my clients have shared the following twenty-five mantras, which have helped them break free or turn away from emotional eating. When you get the urge to emotionally eat, repeat one of these phrases to yourself or write it out on a piece of paper ten times.

"Eat to nourish and energize."

"What am I really hungry for?"

"The wise man should consider that health is the greatest of human blessings. Let food be your medicine." —Hippocrates

"I'm in charge of fueling my body mindfully."

"Food is fuel."

"I'm strengthening my 'resistance' muscle. It's getting stronger!"

"Self-care."

"Eat. Real. Food."

"The greatest wealth is health." —Virgil

"The body is like a piano, and happiness is like music. It is needful to have the instrument in good order." —Henry Ward Beecher

"In this food I see the entire universe supporting my existence."

"I practice gratitude with each bite. Gratitude for the farmers who grew the food, for hands that picked it, for drivers who brought it, for clerks who stocked it, for the earth and sun and rain that made it grow."

"What you think you become." —Buddha

"Be the change you wish to see in the world." —Gandhi

"Every day in every way I'm getting better and better." —Laura Silva

"I change my thoughts, I change my world." —Norman Vincent Peale

"I am flexible and flowing."

"My body knows what to do with this food. Trust it."

"Describe the taste. Describe the texture. Describe the feel."

"What do I *really* want?"

"Now is the time. Make mindful choices today!"

"Choose health."

"Peace" on the in-breath, "Presence" on the out-breath.

"Eat, drink, and be mindful." —Susan Albers

"Peace."

Invent Your Own Mantra

Choose a mantra that resonates with you. You can say it to your-self silently or out loud whenever you feel the urge to overeat or emotionally eat. Repeat it to yourself slowly 5 to 10 times. If you are in a bad mood or feeling stressed, which leaves you at risk for emotional eating, try repeating your special phrase to help shift your feelings in a better direction.

I subscribe to my own mantra: eat less, move more, eat plenty of fruits and vegetables, don't eat too much junk food, and enjoy what you eat. Or, to summarize: eat less, eat better, move more, and get political. —Marion Nestle

14. Self-Compassion

I am enough.

I accept myself just as I am.

I am worthy of the same love I give to others.

These are words we don't tell ourselves very often—if ever. Most of us are all too well acquainted with that sneaky, critical inner voice that whispers discouraging and sometimes demeaning things into our ear. Occasionally, it isn't a whisper but a loud roar, sounding more like "Go ahead and eat another cookie—you're fat anyway, it doesn't really matter." This language leads emotional eaters to eat in secrecy and to feel guilty, shameful, and completely out of control. Most of all, self-criticism leads to avoidance—prompting some to do anything to distract, escape, or quiet those awful thoughts.

A 2014 study in the journal *Health Psychology* suggests that there is an important skill that can significantly make or break your efforts to eat healthier: self-compassion (Sirois, Kitner, and Hirsch 2014). In this review of studies on self-compassion and healthy behaviors, the authors suggest that being kind, compassionate, and having an accepting stance toward yourself during difficult times is key to eating well.

My clinical observations confirm what this study suggests. People need a gentle, soothing inner voice to be able to eat well and live better. Why? Basically, people who have self-compassion are able to adapt to and manage their emotions. If they have an "oops, why did I eat that" moment, they can deal with it well without emotionally crumbling. They allow themselves a break (and everyone makes mistakes), and know it's not the end of the world. They don't become overly self-critical, which leads to feeling bad about yourself. When you're frustrated or upset, it can be difficult to make healthy choices. Giving yourself a break helps you bounce back and get right back on track instead of staying stuck in unhealthy emotional eating. In other words, while it isn't easy, it's essential to stop being so hard on yourself!

Another study in the journal of *Psychological Health* found that a compassionate inner voice is necessary to be able to complete food diaries, an important task in improving your overall diet and in taking charge of emotional eating (Mantzios and Wilson 2014). Writing down what you eat, when you eat it, and whether you are emotionally or physically hungry is a great exercise for reducing emotional eating. You will see patterns and changes, and you'll feel more in control of your eating too!

Soothing Strategy
Get the Language

Start with noticing and being mindful of how you talk to yourself. When does the soft, soothing voice come out or the critical one creep in? Then, intentionally use language and phrases that convey compassion: "It's okay" or "You are enough just as you are" or "It will get better, you are doing the best you can." If you don't know what to say, imagine what you would say to a child or a friend who feels bad about something. When your critical voice comes forward, immediately counter it with a kind, compassionate statement.

Soothing Strategy
Become the Scientist

Aren't quite ready to be compassionate? A first step is to put on your scientific hat and investigate. Be curious. Ask yourself "why" questions, gently inquiring why you did what you did. For example, instead of saying "I am such an idiot for overeating!" ask yourself, "What were the factors that led me to overeat?" or "What can I learn from this?"

If you feel that you have a particularly harsh inner critic and want more information on compassion, check out Dr.

Kristin Neff's work at http://www.self-compassion.org or Dr. Christopher Germer's at http://www.mindfulselfcompassion.org.

Soothing Strategy
Send a Letter

Writing a compassionate letter to oneself has also been shown to improve coping with life events and general well-being (Germer and Neff 2013). When you are feeling the urge to emotionally eat, write a letter to yourself empathizing with this urge to eat. Also, at the end of each day you can jot down a few compassionate words in a diary. This will help lift your mood overall.

Soothing Strategy
Compassion Meditation

When you are in need of some compassion to counteract the inner critic, you will find this exercise particularly helpful. You can also practice it regularly to help this calm and gentle way of being come to mind more frequently.

- Place two hands on your lips and say to yourself, "May I be more mindful of my words and speak with compassion and kindness."

- Place your two hands over your heart and say to yourself, "May I be more mindful of my feelings and send out compassion to myself and others."

- Clasp your hands gently together and say to yourself, "May the things I do show kindness and compassion for myself and others."

I have just three things to teach: simplicity, patience, compassion. These three are your greatest treasures. —Lao Tzu

Mindful Breathing

Many of my clients are not sure how altering their breathing habits will ultimately help them manage emotion and their eating. They balk when I suggest deep breathing, as though it's a lame solution and too undemanding to be effective. In all honesty, slow, deep breathing can make you feel more relaxed. Try it right now. Take a deep breath and see what happens. A large, slow breath. Tune in to your mind and body. What happens? Although you can feel the soothing result, you might think that it doesn't seem complicated enough as a technique to change your behavior, right? The purpose of this chapter is to show you that mindful breathing can make a signficant positive impact on your stress level and your relationship to comfort eating. And, as you've just experienced, it's easy to do!

Some of the breathing techniques might be hard to visualize, and you might be wondering if you're practicing them correctly. To see how each of the following breathing exercises are done, watch me demonstrate at http://www.eatingmindfully.com/demonstrations.

15. Abdominal Breathing

Do you know that when you are feeling anxious or a high level of stress you're most likely breathing through your chest? Chest breathing is generally quick and shallow. When you are relaxed, you breathe more diaphragmatically, from the abdomen. These breaths tend to be longer and slower. Think of what a dog looks like when basking in the sun or a baby when sleeping; the belly moves up and down in a slow, rhythmic movement.

Diaphragmatic breathing increases the amount of oxygen to the body and is the perfect antidote to anxiety because it interrupts the natural fight-or-flight response and triggers the relaxation response.

I often prescribe this technique to my clients, particularly those who are comfort eaters. A simple switch in the way they breathe makes a big difference in their anxiety levels. Jane, for example, needed a mobile option for calming her nerves before board exams in nursing school. Not only did she turn to chronic snacking while studying; she wanted snacks while taking her test. But when test time came, she found herself without the crutch she had become dependent on. Teaching Jane these abdominal breathing exercises has made all the difference in her stress levels. Now she can practice them at home, while studying, and even during exams. She's eliminated a lot of her mindless eating habits.

Take the following steps before, during, or after any stressful events or when you find yourself wanting to eat for comfort.

Lie on the floor or sit upright in a chair with both feet on the ground. Place both hands on your abdominal area. As you inhale, let your belly expand into your hands. As you exhale, let your belly button drop toward your spine.

Focus on long, slow breaths, breathing in through your nose and out through your nose. If your nose is clogged, breathe in through your mouth, but make sure that you are breathing slowly and deeply. Take 6 to 12 breaths, making the exhalations a little longer than the inhalations. The longer your exhalations, the quieter your mind will get. Conversely, to increase energy, focus on slightly longer inhalations.

What we call "I" is just a swinging door, which moves when we inhale and when we exhale. —Shunryu Suzuki

16. Alternate-Nostril Breathing

The ancient practice of *nadi shodhana pranayama*, or alternate-nostril breathing, is basically exactly what it sounds like: breathing through one nostril and then the other in a slow and rhythmic way. The word *nadi* means "subtle energy channel," *shodhana* means "cleaning" or "purification," and *pranayama* means "breathing technique." Although it may sound or look a little funny, research has shown that this technique decreases blood pressure; increases skin conductivity, or the sympathetic nervous system; and decreases heart rate (Telles, Sharma, and Balkrishna 2014; Raghuraj and Telles 2008). Breathing out of the left nostril induces calmness, empathy, sensitivity, and cleansing energy, while breathing out of the right nostril promotes concentration, alertness, and willpower. In fact, alternating nostrils provides a combination of excellent benefits to help with comfort eating.

Interestingly, an Indian study found that this form of yogic breathing helped to lower blood pressure, pulse rate, and respiratory rate for thirty-six volunteers who followed a four-week program of alternate-nostril breathing for fifteen minutes per day each morning on an empty stomach (Turankar et al. 2013). It's an excellent way to calm and center your mind, as it actually helps to balance the left and right brain.

Breathing into the right nostril brings oxygen to the right hemisphere of the brain, responsible for the creative brain governing rhythm, spatial awareness, color, imagination, daydreaming, and holistic awareness. Breathing into the left nostril brings oxygen into the left hemisphere of the brain, which is the logical brain responsible for words, logic, numbers, analysis, lists, and sequence. And like all the breathing practices, bringing more oxygen into the system is excellent for your energy and thinking. My clients often experience alternate-nostril breathing as a "cleansing" breath, one that helps them to clear out the urge to emotionally eat.

When you feel confused or overwhelmed, try alternate-nostril breathing. It will help you feel grounded, centered, and focused. Follow these steps for alternate-nostril breathing:

- Sit upright in a chair with both feet on the ground.

- Bending your right elbow, place the tips of your right index and middle fingers in between your eyebrows. Then place your right thumb on your right nostril. Close your right nostril as you inhale through the left.

- At the top of the inhalation, close the left nostril with the ring finger of your hand, release the right thumb, and exhale through the right nostril. Then inhale through the right nostril.

- At the top of the inhalation, close the right nostril with your thumb, release your ring finger, and exhale through the left. This is 1 round.

- It is best to practice with your eyes closed. Focus on long, slow breaths.

- Perform 6 to 12 rounds. Then rest for a moment with your eyes closed when you are finished, noticing the quality of your mind and emotions.

Feelings come and go like clouds in a windy sky. Conscious breathing is my anchor. —Thich Nhat Hanh

17. Left-Nostril Breathing

Did you know that you tend to naturally breathe out of one nostril at a time and then switch automatically in a repeated cycle? This cycle was first studied in 1895 by a German nose doctor, Richard Kayser. He discovered that your breath can have a tremendous impact on your body chemistry and how the brain functions. What's more, one-nostril breathing has been shown to change your metabolism, and this could help you actually burn more calories from the foods you eat (Pal et al. 2014).

Left-nostril breathing is particularly helpful when you have trouble falling asleep or wake up in the middle of the night and can't quickly return to dreamland. Of course, you can also use left-nostril breathing anytime you're anxious, worried, or stressed out, especially before public speaking, giving a presentation, or taking any kind of test. A study of men and women twenty to forty-five years old showed that the participants exhibited increased spatial math skills and improved cognition after practicing left-nostril breathing, making it not only a calming solution but an excellent prework exercise too (Joshi and Telles 2008).

Your cravings or emotions don't have to control you. Even out your feelings by learning how to control your breath. It is a powerful ally! Here's how you do it:

- If in bed, lie on your right side. Or sit upright in a chair with both feet on the ground.

- Place your right thumb over you right nostril and close it.

- Begin to breathe in and out of your left nostril. If you find that your left nostril is clogged, then skip this breath and practice one of the others in this section.

- If using this technique to fall asleep, take 26 breaths; if sitting in a chair, take 6 to 12 breaths.

- Focus on long, slow breaths, making the exhalation a little longer than the inhalation.

When you own your breath, nobody can steal your peace.
—Anonymous

18. Skull-Shining Breath

Kapalabhati, or skull-shining breath, improves focus and concentration, and helps release toxins from the body (Telles et al. 2011). It also helps you to feel more alert and energized, and it clears your mind. If you do a lot of boredom eating, you'll find this technique particularly effective.

About 80 percent of the toxins in our body are released through the outgoing breath, so kapalabhati is said to detoxify, improve metabolism, increase blood circulation, bring radiance to the face, and rejuvenate brain cells. The cognitive benefits of kapalabhati have actually been studied in clinical research. A 2009 study in the *Journal of Alternative and Complementary Medicine* gave subjects one of two tasks. They either practiced kapalabhati at the speed of two exhalations per second for one minute, or they were placed in a breath-awareness group. Both groups were given a challenging mental task before and after the breathing exercise. The study showed that practicing skull-shining breath improved mental performance on cognitive tasks (Joshi and Telles 2009).

Kapalabhati also helps *perceived stress*, which is one way of explaining how some people are more affected by stress than others. One study looked at the perceived stress and cardiovascular function of young health care workers. Participants practiced both fast and slow kapalabhati breathing. Both forms showed significant improvement in their perceived stress and related cardiovascular functions (Sharma et al. 2013).

Skull-shining breath is a great pick-me-up and clears the mind of unwanted thoughts. Try it instead of a cup of coffee! Here's how:

Sit upright in a chair with your feet on the ground.

Place your hands on your belly.

Inhale three-fourths of the way through your nose and then exhale sharply through your nostrils the rest of the way, using your hands to help press your belly in toward your spine. This is 1 round. Practice a few rounds and then try it without your hands until you have a feel for this breathing practice.

Now perform a quick series of 20 to 30 breaths. At the end of the last exhale, inhale three-fourths of the way and hold your breath for a few seconds, and then exhale slowly. This is 1 round. Go ahead and do a second round of 20 to 30 breaths.

If at any time you get out of breath, stop and let your breath return to normal. Then begin again. *Caution:* If you have asthma or any lung disorders, do not practice this breath.

Smile, breathe, and go slowly. —T h i c h N h a t H a n h

19. Cooling Breath

Anger is one of the most significant triggers of emotional eating, and many of us actually feel very hot when experiencing it. This is where the expressions "hot under the collar" and "chill out" come from. You can find a way to cool down and relax without reaching for comfort food. You can do it very intentionally with the following basic breathing technique.

Shitali literally means "cooling" in Sanskrit. *Shitali pranayama* is the perfect breath for when you want to tone down angry thoughts and feelings or are simply feeling warm, like in super-hot weather. It's said to lower blood pressure and even help with ulcers. Another great benefit of *shitali pranayama* is that it helps reduce hunger. It works to reduce stomach acidity and improve digestion. Because of this, it's said to take away hunger and thirst.

The purpose of the cooling breath is to reduce the body temperature. When you cool down the temperature of the body, you're more relaxed. Think of a time when you were wound up. It's likely you began stripping off layers of clothing. According to psychological research, the most fights and arrests tend to occur in urban areas on hot days (Bushman, Wang, and Anderson 2005). Heat increases irritability.

Nothing makes my clients grumpier than hot flashes. My client Irene uses the cooling breath to help reduce her irritability when she is experiencing uncomfortable waves of heat in her body. Initially, she was frustrated that she couldn't control what was happening to her own body. At age fifty-five, she noticed herself emotionally eating for the first time, and it was harder than ever to keep her weight stable. The slightest bit of over-eating seemed to make the needle on the scale move up. Now, instead of comfort eating when feeling hot and uncomfortable, she uses the cooling breath technique to feel better fast.

Remember that anger is a natural emotion that we all experience from time to time. The goal is to learn to control it, rather than letting it control you. These breathing practices are great tools for putting the flames out on anger and preventing eating out of irritation, rage, or annoyance.

How to Practice Shitali Pranayama, or Cooling Breath

This breath requires you to curl your tongue into a tube, which is genetically determined—some people can and some can't. If you are one of those who can't, a great alternative breath called *sitari pranayama* is described in the section after this one. To practice *shitari pranayama*:

Extend your tongue past your lips about a half inch and then curl your tongue as if creating a small tube.

Draw in air through your tongue, allowing your belly to expand as you inhale.

Hold the breath in for 5 seconds and then release slowly through your nose. This is 1 round.

Practice 6 to 12 rounds and work up to 20 over time.

How to Practice Sitari Pranayama

Bring your upper and lower jaw together so that your teeth are touching.

With your mouth closed, press your tongue to your teeth.

Keeping your mouth closed, open your lips and slowly draw in air over your tongue, making a hissing sound. Hold for 5 seconds, then slowly exhale through your nose. This is 1 round. If you have trouble drawing in air, release some of the pressure of your tongue against your teeth.

Practice 6 to 12 rounds and work up to 20 over time.

Just by breathing deeply on your anger, you will calm it.
—Thich Nhat Hanh

Alternative Therapies

Alternative therapies have been around for ages, and these timeless practices have been used not only to combat emotional eating but also to restore balance, tranquility, and peace of mind to those who practice them. What are alternative and integrative medicine therapies? For the purposes of this book, I define them as techniques that you can use in lieu of or in conjunction with conventional Western medicine as a way to effectively deal with emotional eating patterns.

Many of these therapies date back to ancient times, and various cultures and societies have met with success by embracing these valuable techniques. For example, the Chinese began identifying acupuncture points and energy meridians in the body more than 2,000 years ago. And the ancient Greeks and Egyptians are said to have used sunlight for therapeutic purposes in people suffering from various diseases. One Taoist practice uses what is termed the "inner smile" to clear negative emotions and the related physical symptoms (by visualizing a smiling energy source that emanates throughout the body to specifically vulnerable body sites such as the heart, lungs, liver, and spleen). And many of our ancestors understood the importance of maintaining our connection with the earth by literally and figuratively "grounding" themselves to remain present in the moment and to maintain emotional and physiological balance.

In this section, we'll explore various alternative therapies that pack the most effective punch when it comes to eating and dealing with cravings. For example, you will learn how to curb your cravings through acupressure, acupuncture, and tapping. You'll also learn how light—both natural and artificial—will not only boost your mood but also alter your desire to eat emotionally.

20. Tapping Away Cravings

If you've ever wanted to try acupuncture—the ancient Chinese technique for healing various ailments—but you're not a fan of needles or the expense of a weekly session, then emotional freedom therapy (EFT) may be the perfect technique for you. EFT includes tapping your fingers gently on various parts of the body while focusing on positive thoughts and feelings. Pretty simple, right?

How does EFT work? Similar to acupuncture, EFT is based on Eastern medicine, which stems from the concept of body energy. Likewise, both techniques focus on using specific body sites (acupressure points) and the pathways that connect those points (meridians) to relieve pain, stress, and inflammation. Honest, it's easier than it sounds.

The EFT technique dates back to the 1980s when a clinical psychologist, Dr. Roger Callahan, developed a type of acupressure called Thought Field Therapy (TFT). EFT then grew out of Dr. Callahan's pioneering work. From a psychological perspective, this technique integrates the connection between the mind and body. According to this theory, your energy flows freely when the body is in optimal working condition. However, any type of distress will disrupt or block that energy.

Now, let's apply this mind-body connection to food. We all know how stressful a craving can be, and within the context of EFT, this distress can create energy blockages. Because EFT opens up the blocked energy, your cravings and the associated distress will disappear once energy begins to flow freely again.

I asked one of my clients, Sophia, how intense her cravings were on a scale from 1 to 10. She said 25! Sophia's cravings were so powerful that she couldn't imagine *not* giving in to them. I challenged her to give this technique a chance, even though she had already tried many different strategies without success. After a few rounds of doing EFT at home, her cravings dropped from a 25...to a 4!

Many other clients have experienced similar results, since they find it difficult to think about food when they are busy tapping and talking. This is due to the fact that, in addition to the proposed theory of changing your energy level, the activity itself is likely to be very distracting—and therefore it takes your mind off your cravings.

The good news is that clinical research trials have revealed promising results for EFT in reducing food cravings in people who are overweight. In a study conducted by Dr. Peta Stapleton at Griffin University School of Medicine, ninety-six overweight or obese adults were given either the EFT treatment or put on a wait list, which meant they didn't receive the treatment. Four weeks later, the researchers found that cravings in the EFT group diminished after only four two-hour EFT sessions, and they maintained positive results at their six-month follow-ups as well (Stapleton et al. 2013).

Other studies concur. For example, in a study published in *Integrative Medicine: A Clinician's Journal*, researchers taught 216 participants to use the EFT technique to cope with psychological distress and cravings. They assessed the participants two hours after applying the EFT technique themselves and ninety days later. The results? Study participants indicated significant improvement on all of the distress scales including ratings of pain, emotional distress, *and* food cravings (Church and Brooks 2010). EFT can be a quick, interesting, and inexpensive way to address cravings.

Soothing Strategy
Tapping with EFT

In this exercise, you will tap lightly on acupressure points while repeating an affirming, positive statement:

First, identify the strength of your craving on a scale from 1 to 10, with 10 being the most intense.

Choose a "setup" statement that both addresses your cravings and creates a positive thought pattern, such as *I can cope with these cravings because I am mindful,* or *I accept myself as I am, including these cravings.* You may also decide to use this sentence frame to create a customized phrase: *Even though I have experienced* [insert your personal issue]*, I deeply and completely accept myself.* Positive statements like these help release and rewire the underlying negative thoughts and beliefs that you may be holding on to.

Now, locate the "karate chop" part of your hand (the outer side of the palm of your hand—along the edge, between the base of your pinky finger and your wrist). You will begin by tapping this point. *Note:* It does not matter which hand you choose for this exercise.

Use your index and middle fingers of the opposite hand to tap approximately 5 times, lightly but firmly. Some recommend taking one complete inhalation and exhalation as you tap.

Continue tapping the following seven points:

- Between your eyebrows (by the bridge of your nose)

- The side of the eye (near the outer corner of your eye socket, on the bone)

- Under the eye (the bony part of the socket that is underneath the eye)

- Under the nose (between your nostrils and upper lip)

- The chin (between your lower lip and chin)

- The collarbone (approximately 1 inch below the U-shaped part of your sternum, where your collarbone, sternum, and first rib meet)

- Under the arm (about 4 inches below the armpit)

As you tap, repeat your chosen setup statement.

After you complete the tapping sequence, revisit the strength of your cravings on a scale of 1 to 10. Did the level drop?

If not, repeat the sequence, always beginning by tapping the karate chop side of your hand. Continue this progression until your desire to give in to your craving has been eliminated.

It is possible that other issues may surface as you use this technique. For instance, maybe an important relationship in your life is causing you stress that is contributing to your cravings. If that's the case, be sure to create statements that address those issues as well so that you can try to lessen your cravings. And for those of you seeking more support, there are EFT practitioners who can assist you in fine-tuning your practice.

Everybody has their own way of tapping into their realness.
—Sandra Bernhard

21. Acupuncture and Acupressure Points

Many medical professionals have now realized the benefits of this ancient alternative therapy. In fact, did you know that acupuncture is available at the top medical facilities in the world today? And as this therapy has become more and more common, health insurance companies have gotten on board to cover this treatment method. You may also be able to find clinics in some cities where the fees are very low.

Traditional Chinese medicine describes acupuncture as a 2,000-year-old practice that works on the body's life energy or *qi* (pronounced "chee"). The tiny acupuncture needles are thought to release blockages at various points in the body's qi that help release the life energy to flow freely, restoring good health, reducing pain, and helping with emotional issues such as emotional eating.

Modern science theorizes that acupuncture needles release endorphins into our body that have the same chemical structure as morphine or opiates, reducing pain and helping with other health issues.

I once counseled a forty-two-year-old woman who was struggling while serving as a caregiver to her parents and sister. She was exhausted and depressed, and worried about her health. First, she tried treating her depression with medication, which she found moderately helpful. But after several months of acupuncture treatment, her urge to eat emotionally dropped significantly, she reported feeling less depressed, and she found she had more energy—results that medication didn't seem to deliver. In retrospect, she attributes her improvement to counseling and the acupuncture treatment, along with making herself more of a priority than she had in the past.

If you don't have access to an acupuncture therapist, or if you find it is too expensive—or if you simply are in need of relief *right now* in your battle with food—you can do what is called *acupressure*. Like acupuncture, acupressure applies gentle pressure to specific points on the body to promote healing. It can be self-applied and works on the same theory that stimulating various trigger points on the body can release endorphins or qi to help heal.

There are many ways you can do acupressure, but I am going to focus on two simple techniques that specifically deal with weight loss and soothing your emotions.

Soothing Skill
Try a Gua Sha Treatment

Spoon away your stress not in a bowl but on your face. If you need to feel a moment of calm and distraction, try this ancient Chinese treatment. And if you need a demonstration, visit http://www.eatingmindfully.com/demonstrations.

Apply a light cream, such as a daily moisturizer, all over your face.

Hold a clean spoon vertical to your nose and with its curved side facing you. Now give it a quarter turn and apply its edge to your forehead's midline.

Begin to stroke the spoon's edge upward and outward from mid-forehead to your hairline above your left eyebrow. Apply firm but not painful pressure. Do this 12 times.

Then repeat 12 strokes above your right eyebrow.

Next, return to the left side, but begin the stroke lower on the forehead, sweeping upward and outward to your hairline. Repeat 12 times on both sides.

Next, complete two sets of 12 strokes across the cheeks on both sides, then two more sets of 12 strokes under the chin on both sides of the face.

Soothing Strategy
Acupressure for Weight Management

This acupressure technique targets addictions, obesity, and inflammation. It is based on applying pressure to the part of the ear called the "Heavenly Gate." The Heavenly Gate is the upper region of the outer ear, which is the body site most closely linked to weight loss. This pressure point was discovered in research conducted by a French physician, Dr. Paul Nogier, in 1956, after he observed that a patient's backache disappeared after his ear was burned.

A Korean research study (Yeo, Kim, and Lim 2013) also supports this technique for weight loss, as researchers found that using acupuncture on the ear helped people reduce their body mass index (BMI) more than those who had a placebo treatment (in which the acupuncture needles were removed immediately after insertion).

Practitioners who have utilized this pressure point for acupuncture and acupressure have been successful in treating drug addictions, smoking addictions, and weight loss (Fogarty et al. 2015).

In this version of acupressure, simply apply pressure to your outer ear by pressing firmly and moving your finger in a circular motion. Or, you may wish to massage the area by pinching it from either side, with your thumb on one side of the ear and your index and middle finger on the other. With either technique, apply the pressure for approximately 30 to 60 seconds.

Soothing Strategy
Acupressure to Soothe Emotions

If your emotions are getting the best of you—and therefore tempting you with food cravings—soothe yourself with this exercise that focuses on what is termed the "Great Mount" of your hand (also known as "Pericardium 7"):

> Find the spot located in the middle of the inside wrist (found in the dip between the two tendons, on or just below the crease of the wrist).

> Rub your finger gently (with light pressure) in a counter-clockwise direction on this point. Continue for about 10 turns. *Note:* If you prefer, you can use a pencil eraser to apply gentle pressure.

One of the great benefits of acupressure and acupuncture is that you can easily track your progress. For instance, if you are feeling anxious, note your level of anxiety on a scale from 1 to 10 before and after your acupressure or acupuncture session. It may be even more helpful to note your scores in a journal, so you can look for trends and improvements over time.

When we long for a life without difficulties, remind us that oaks grow strong in contrary winds and diamonds are made under pressure. —Peter Marshall

22. Light Therapy

The majority of my clients live in Northeast Ohio, but I receive letters and e-mails from readers who live in frigid places, from Alaska to Iceland. Therefore, every year, when fall comes to an end and winter begins, some of my clients begin to show signs of SAD (seasonal affective disorder). As the name reflects, SAD is a condition in which sufferers exhibit symptoms of sadness or depression about the same time each year, usually when it's cold and there are fewer daylight hours. I've also noticed that as the temperatures drop, clients and readers begin to report a dramatic increase in emotional eating as well. It's no surprise that people who are sensitive to the cold and darkness tend to eat more carbohydrates and sweets during the winter (Danilenko et al. 2008).

The question is, does the weather have something do to with the increase in eating? Definitely. First, the sunlight itself has a lot to do with the way we eat. Your body runs on a clock that is set by the sun. That makes sense, when you think about this from a biological perspective. Before electric lights, the sun was society's first alarm clock, setting our wake and sleep cycles.

Being cooped up in the house doesn't help, either; you may feel cramped up, penned in, or isolated from others in a way that you don't experience in the spring and summer months. Certainly, those feelings of being alone could contribute to emotional eating, too. Not to mention the sheer fact that you are in close proximity to the kitchen!

Today, we have the luxury of "ignoring" the sun, since we set schedules based on externally imposed agendas; however, our bodies still rely on light and heat to set our internal clocks. Unfortunately, our ability to schedule events independent of daylight doesn't mean our bodies have adapted.

In addition to helping your mood, a recently published study has revealed that bright lights in the morning reduced body fat and appetite in a group of women struggling with their weight (Danilenko, Mustafina, and Pechenkina 2013). In this study, thirty-four overweight women ages twenty to fifty-four from Novosibirsk, Russia, tried light therapy for three weeks (versus a placebo group that was exposed to an ion light). At the end, the women had a lower percentage of fat, fat mass, and appetite. It makes sense. We feel better in the light and are more motivated to eat well when we feel good! How interesting that this intervention only required the addiction of light therapy—not calories, exercise, or anything else.

Hopefully, you are beginning to see the important role that light can play in your life when it comes to weight, mood, and your propensity to eat for emotional reasons. The exercises below address both ends of this sunlight spectrum by suggesting ways to get more light early in the day—and less at night.

Soothing Strategy
Lights Out for Soothing Sleep

- **Make your room as dark as possible.** When you're ready to catch some Zs, turn off the television and computer, draw the shades or curtains, and turn off any other artificial lights. If there are lights on in other parts of your house, be sure to close your bedroom door to block as much light as possible.

- **Turn off your cell phone two hours before you go to bed.** Having it on keeps your brain awake and stimulated. Whether you know it or not, your brain is on alert for getting e-mail or hearing it ring. Also, there are some theories that the light produced by the screen stimulates activity in your brain that may be keeping you awake. If you can't turn it off completely, try this experiment: place the phone at least 6 feet away from your head at night (and facedown to reduce the amount of light the phone emits). The best answer, though, is to charge your phone at night in a separate area away from your sleeping environment, like in the kitchen.

- **Consider a sleep mask.** You might wear a sleep mask over your eyes to block out all light, especially if you leave a hall light on for other family members, or if there's any other light in your sleeping environment that can't be eliminated.

Soothing Strategy
Light Up Your Life...With Light Therapy

Even if you don't live in a perennially sunny climate, you can trick your mind into feeling like it's basking in the sun with artificial light therapy. Many companies now manufacture lights, lamps, and light boxes that mimic the sun's rays, and you can simply flick these lights on in the morning to give your body the light that it's seeking. Some companies that specialize in this type of lighting include Verilux, Northern Light Technologies, NatureBright, and Caribbean Sun. Read the directions for time recommendations for your light therapy sessions, as they may vary from several minutes to several hours each day.

Be sure to use the lights earlier in the day. Then, once you get a sense of your body's reaction to the therapy, you can monitor how late in the day you can keep the lights on without affecting your nighttime sleep. Also, be cognizant of the length of time you expose yourself to this light during a session. Some people report that if they keep the lights on too long—even early in the day—they have difficulty sleeping at night. Just remember to keep everything in moderation so that you can balance your body's need for nighttime darkness with its craving for light in the morning.

Soothing Strategy
Bask in Natural Light

Take advantage of natural sunlight as much as possible, even if you don't live in the sunniest climate. Get outside in the early morning hours when you let your dog out, take a 10-minute walk during your lunch break, or fit in a jog right after work (if there's still daylight at that time). Even enjoying the sunlight on a ski slope can work! Any opportunity to expose your body to natural light is beneficial, and if you can allow the vitamin D from the sun's rays to shine on your skin (arms, face, and so on), that's even better. Of course, be sure to take intelligent precautions with sunscreen, and don't overdo the exposure if your body isn't used to it.

Keep your face always toward the sunshine—and shadows will fall behind you. —Walt Whitman

23. Rituals

Imagine sitting down for dinner, lighting a few candles, setting the table with cloth napkins and fine china, and then artfully arranging your food on the plate. Conversely, imagine yourself getting ready for the same meal, but without the thoughtful preparations and routines. Do you think your food enjoyment would be any different between these two hypothetical situations? If you had to choose which dining experience would be more enjoyable, chances are you'd select the first scenario.

But why? Is it the fine china? The ambience created when eating by candlelight? The aesthetic appreciation of the food presentation?

If you think about it, the first scene has nothing to do with the food itself—the cut of meat, the freshness of the produce, or the flavor of the foods. Instead, it is the set of behaviors surrounding the experience that makes the difference. And if those behaviors (candlelight, food arrangement, and so forth) are typical ones, then this could be considered a ritual—a habitual set of behaviors that are performed in a particular order and linked to a certain set of circumstances (in this case, dinner). This is important to consider, because by adopting rituals, you may be able to enhance your eating experience—and decrease your tendency to eat for emotional reasons.

An interesting study revealed that enacting a ritual around your food can not only heighten your enjoyment of the food; it can also result in improved portion control, a slower pace of eating, and even a willingness to pay more for the food you're eating (Vohs et al. 2013). Now, before you think that this study examined only fine-dining experiences or highly desirable foods, you may be surprised to find that was not the case; in fact, the researchers, believe it or not, used rituals to help people increase their anticipation for eating baby carrots (Vohs et al. 2013)! Think for a moment of the types of food rituals you have—maybe you cut your sandwich the same direction every day, or eat a combination of tomato soup and grilled cheese, or drink out of your favorite mug on Sunday mornings. These types of rituals are comforting.

Behavioral routines can also provide you with quite a bit of comfort. One client, Shirley, fills her favorite glass with water and ice cubes before she goes to bed. Even when she goes on vacation, she brings that particular glass, because following that nighttime ritual to a tee helps her fall asleep. She is lost without it. Other clients talk about comforting sequences of getting ready in the morning. Shannon, a college student, tells me that her routine is breakfast, shower, and reading her e-mail—in that order exactly. When she oversleeps and runs to class, her entire day is thrown off, causing her to feel like she is in disarray. In other words, don't underestimate the power and comfort of shifting into a routine. What's interesting about this is that you can establish or set up a healthy routine that, with repetition, will provide significant comfort.

Right now, get out a piece of paper. Take a few minutes to consider whether you already have any comfort routines in place.

Do you have a nighttime or morning ritual? Is there something you do when you are having a bad day? Maybe you treat yourself with a cup of gourmet coffee, or go to bed at 9:00? Be clear on these routines, because often they are so automatic that you no longer realize you are doing them. They're simply ingrained.

Soothing Strategy
Leaving Your Troubles at the Door

Have you heard the saying about leaving your troubles at the door? This refers to not bringing your concerns wherever you go. If you're someone who starts emotionally eating the moment you enter the front door as a way to unwind from the day, make it a ritual to take your shoes off before you enter your home. Do it slowly and mindfully. As you take off the shoes, say to yourself, "I leave my troubles here." Repeat this ritual daily whenever you return and enter your home. Create a new routine. If you typically head to the kitchen to read the mail and grab a snack, go into the bedroom instead, change out of work clothes, plop down in a comfy chair, and read the mail. You've created a new routine.

Soothing Strategy
Create a Soothing Ritual

Choose one of the following times to create a new ritual that works for *you*. Let's say you have difficulty falling asleep. Perhaps you decide on a wind-down ritual to look like this: Stretch, journal for 5 minutes, read for 20 minutes, then lights out. Repeat this sequence for two weeks. What will you notice? After repetition of a particular activity, carrying it out becomes comforting. Imagine how you can use this to help you when you feel stressed out. Moving into a set sequence of behaviors may help. Come up with a few rituals following various times in your day:

Nighttime

Morning

Snack time

Stressful moments

Soothing Strategy
Creating Your Personal Eating Ritual

If you create a ritual for your mealtimes, you'll be able to start fully enjoying your food, become more conscious of what you're eating, increase the odds of controlling your portions, and even slow down the rate at which you eat. Here's how:

First, determine which meal you would like to begin with when it comes to establishing a ritual. Choose a time of day when you're most likely to eat in the same place—and perhaps even the same time, which will increase consistency.

Next, consider how much time you normally allot for this meal, and decide how much additional time you have to create a ritual around your eating. The ritual need not be overly time-consuming; even a minute or two can be enough for a meaningful ritual.

Decide upon a behavior or set of behaviors that you would like to establish as your personal ritual. Maybe you want to arrange your food in a certain way on the plate; maybe you want to dim the lights, play special music, or use special utensils and plates; or maybe you want to say a prayer of gratitude before you begin eating. Whatever you decide, make sure it's something you find meaningful, enjoyable, and realistic for your daily schedule.

After several days of implementing the new ritual, take note of any changes in your feelings surrounding this meal. Are you enjoying the food more? Is the flavor enhanced? Are you able to eat less because you enjoy it more? Are certain "healthy" foods that you don't normally enjoy now more palatable to you?

The modern habit of doing ceremonial things unceremoniously is no proof of humility; rather it proves the offender's inability to forget himself in the rite, and his readiness to spoil for everyone else the proper pleasure of ritual. —C.S. Lewis

Mindful Movement

While movement is important, the kind that I am presenting in this section is what I refer to as "mindful movement." Mindful movement is paying attention to the sensations of movement and being truly *in* your body while you're doing it. For example, it's likely you've had the experience of dancing at a party. A song that you love starts to play. Suddenly, your dancing takes on a different form and energy. You dance a little faster, your movements are more in sync with the music, and you really enjoy it. Some forms of movement, like paddle boarding and rock climbing, demand more mindfulness than others. You can't be thinking about anything else. You have to be mentally present while doing it—or else you won't be successful at it and you will fall or get hurt! Other types of exercise don't require that you be mentally present—aerobics, for example. You can mindlessly jump around without much mental effort. Doing exercise mindlessly may be why sometimes people find movement boring or don't get a lot out of it. So when you do move, I challenge you to do it mindfully.

While there are many forms of movement therapy, the following modalities have special value to those dealing with emotional eating: Tai Chi, Pilates, self-massage, and mudras. Note that mudras are not necessarily a movement form; however, they use the body (hands) to connect to the mind, resulting in some unique benefits. I recommend that you review them all, sampling the activities in each section and seeing which ones you are drawn to. Remember, we have bodies and are born to move!

24. Tai Chi

If you are looking to reduce stress, Tai Chi is ranked high in CAM (complementary and alternative techniques) options because it is so effective and can be done by just about anyone. Tai Chi is an ancient Chinese art of gentle movement and exercise that evolved out of a self-defense method (sometimes called shadow boxing) into slow, flowing, graceful actions that provide stress relief while encouraging mindfulness and a deeper connection with the body. It's gentle and noncompetitive, and it can be done at your own pace. The benefits Tai Chi promises are extensive:

- Improved blood flow and circulation

- Strengthened immune system, minimized risk of illness

- Reduced congestive heart failure symptoms

- Lowered blood pressure and cholesterol levels

- Increased balance, reduced risk of falling in older adults

- Higher quality of sleep

- Reduced joint pain and inflammation associated with arthritis

- Reduced gastrointestinal symptoms such as colitis, ulcers, and irritable bowel (Li, Yuan, and Zhang 2014)

Tai Chi is particularly attractive to people who know exercise will help ease their stress level but don't really enjoy exercising. I have many clients who say things like, "I don't like to sweat" or "I *hate* exercise." The flowing, graceful, and slow movements of Tai Chi don't trigger the stress that complicated cardio or aerobic classes can. For this reason, it is often something that many of my clients like and enjoy, even if they don't like traditional exercise.

Tai Chi, in contrast to some of the other CAM techniques, is one that has quite a lot of clinical research to back it up. This may be due to the longevity of the technique or because there are structured poses and programs for teaching the techniques. For example, a review of twenty-one Tai Chi control trials—control trials, incidentally, are the most helpful studies—that included more than 2,100 participants between them, found significant improvements in health-related quality of life for those who participated in Tai Chi (Li, Yuan, and Zhang 2014).

One group of clients I work with who particularly struggle with emotional eating are those diagnosed with fibromyalgia, a condition that causes chronic pain and fatigue. When you are in pain, you often turn to food to help get immediate comfort. Tai Chi has been particularly helpful to these patients in dealing with the pain. Whether reducing smoking or food cravings, Tai Chi has been helpful in managing longings for food or other substances, resulting in weight loss (Dechamps et al. 2009).

When you feel the urge to comfort eat, try one of the following Tai Chi poses for 5 minutes.

Soothing Strategy
Pouring Pose

This Tai Chi stance is helpful in deactivating stress and intentionally calming the mind and body. Use it when waiting in line starts to cause frustration. Maybe you're standing in a grocery store line behind someone who doesn't have a tag on an item. Or you're standing in the hallway listening to your coworker rant about a project. Being captive in a standing position can lead to stress on the body and the mind. You can use this time to actively and intentionally calm yourself. Here's how:

Place both feet flat on the floor, shoulder width apart.

Very slowly shift all of your weight to your right side and right leg. As you do this, imagery may help. Imagine each leg to be like a glass. You pour everything from one glass to the other, slowly, filling up one side and leaving the other empty. You are in charge.

Once all your weight is distributed on one side, hold for 5 seconds.

While holding, allow this side to be completely full, and the other side completely empty and light.

Pour back to center. Hold for 5 seconds.

Repeat to the left side, gently pouring until "full."

Continue pouring from side to side. Don't forget to breathe.

Soothing Strategy
Shooting the Bow

This Tai Chi exercise is good for letting go of and releasing tension.

Stand with your feet shoulder width apart. Bend your knees and round your back slightly. Look straight ahead of you.

Make a fist with both palms and put them directly in front of your face. Your fingers should be facing you and the sides of your palms touching.

Pivot at the waist and turn to your left.

Extend your left hand in front of you and open up your palm facing out. Your right arm should move back as if shooting an arrow from a bow.

Say or imagine letting go of something. It might be an emotion. It may be something stressful that you have been holding on to. Say to yourself, "I let it go."

Repeat as many times as needed.

Bend and you will be whole. Curl and you will be straight. Keep empty and you will be filled. Grow old and you will be renewed.
—Tao Te Ching

25. Mudras

Hand mudras are finger positions or hand gestures that stimulate different types of consciousness. They can be used by themselves or in conjunction with meditation or *pranayama* (yogic breathing exercises). Mudras often include curling, crossing, stretching, or touching your hands and fingers together in various ways. To illustrate how powerful finger positions can be, consider these common gestures of our modern society: thumbs up, thumbs down, the middle finger, the index finger and thumb joined to mean "okay," and the index finger pointing or being held up to get someone's attention.

If you've ever taken a yoga class or have seen pictures of Buddha or yogis, you may notice that their hands are not gently folded in their lap but rather positioned in interesting and sometimes complex ways. This isn't just for decoration. The point of the mudras is to guide your mind and body to various states of consciousness, such as relaxation, improving energy to release guilt, attracting wealth, and enhancing your relationships.

Indeed, the mudras promise many health benefits including everything from healing physical problems to working out emotional issues. A paper published by the National Academy of Sciences showed that hand gestures work to change your mood because they stimulate the same regions in the brain as language. At the University of Pennsylvania, researchers found that doing a Kundalini yoga practice called Kirtan Kriya, which includes mudras, for twelve minutes daily for eight weeks led to an improvement in clarity, empathy, emotional equilibrium, and memory (Newberg et al. 2010; Khalsa et al. 2009).

Many of my clients use mudras to keep their hands occupied and away from food; they also find that using them helps create a sense of calm and balance. Another benefit of mudras is that they can be done anywhere at any time. Try out these ancient hand movements to heal modern stressors right now!

Soothing Strategy
Kundalini Mudra

You'll find that this mudra can help you to be calm and to concentrate. It is especially helpful when you're feeling stressed or need to keep your hands busy instead of reaching for snacks. It's something you can do sitting down, lying down, standing, walking, or while you are talking. Practice for 5 minutes at a time throughout the day.

Touch the tips of your thumbs to the tips of your index fingers. Say to yourself, "Calm and concentrate."

Touch the tips of your thumbs to the tips of your middle fingers. Say to yourself, "Patience."

Touch the tips of your thumbs to the tips of your ring fingers. Say to yourself, "Energy, stability, and self-confidence."

Touch the tips of your thumbs to the tips of your pinkie fingers. Say to yourself, "Intuition and feeling."

Soothing Strategy
Vayu Mudra

This mudra is very helpful when you are feeling upset or impatient.

Start with open palms. Bend your index fingers in toward your palms until the tips touch the palm. Next, touch your thumbs to the first knuckle of the index fingers. Then extend the other three fingers. Rest the backs of your hands on your knees or thighs.

Say to yourself, "I am calm right here and now."

Repeat 5 times.

Soothing Strategy
Uttarabodhi Mudra

Making healthy food decisions isn't always easy. Before deciding what to eat, take a moment to do this mudra, as it will help make a decision or take you out of indecision. Uttarabodhi mudra is also good for settling overexcited nerves.

Interlace your fingers together in front of your navel, thumbs facing your body.

Next, extend your index fingers up and your thumbs down. Bring the tips of the index fingers together and the tips of the thumbs together. Your index fingers and thumbs should now create a diamond shape.

Hold for 5 to 15 minutes. You can also experiment combining this mudra with a meditation practice.

Soothing Strategy
Prana Mudra

Sometimes a lack of energy or a run-down feeling can lead to emotional eating. Instead of reaching for unhealthy, calorie-laden snacks, use prana mudra. This mudra is rejuvenating and helps to improve the immune system.

To practice prana mudra, bring the tips of your thumbs together with the tips of your ring and pinkie fingers. Extend the index and middle fingers. Rest the back of your hands on your lap or knees with palms up. Practice five to ten minutes. For best results, combine with a meditation practice.

The hand is the visible part of the brain. —Immanuel Kant

26. Self-Massage

In addition to reducing stress, triggering deep relaxation, and relieving muscle tension, the benefits of massage are many, including being helpful for anxiety, digestive disorders, headaches, insomnia, myofascial pain, nerve pain, soft tissue sprains and strains, injuries, and more (Field 2014). On an emotional level, massage also helps with depression, anger, grief work, releasing pent-up energy, improving the connection to yourself and others, and helping rewrite emotional patterns and scripts. And for most of us, massage just simply feels great!

While massages by a professional massage therapist can be the ultimate splurge in relaxation, massages can do a number on your wallet, and they just aren't handy when you really need them. Dialing up your favorite masseuse isn't going to cut it when you're in the middle of a chocolate craving.

But don't worry if you don't have time to book an appointment or don't have the extra funds for a massage. Self-massage is the perfect answer. In fact, you may already be doing some self-massage and not even realizing it; when stressed, most of us tend to naturally rub our temples or feet in an effort to feel better and release tension. Self-massage is also a great way to pamper yourself.

Soothing Strategy
Full-Body Self-Massage

This is a great practice when you have a little extra time—and it feels wonderful! It may be best done in the bathroom, as you'll be using oil, and will probably want to shower or bathe afterward. Alternatively, lie on a big, soft bath sheet.

Warm some jojoba or sweet almond oil.

Start by applying oil to the crown of your head and begin to slowly massage your entire scalp.

Put oil on your fingertips and, starting at the neck, begin to make circular motions up your neck and over your entire face including jaws, cheeks, forehead, temples, and ears.

Bring your attention to your arms and legs. On your joints (ankles, knees, elbows, and wrists) use circular motions; on the limbs, use long strokes. Massage from the farthest point away from your heart toward your body.

For the stomach and chest use clockwise, circular motions.

Massage your feet, and be sure to give some attention to your toes.

If possible, sit for a few moments and let the oils absorb into your body. Then take a warm shower or bath. When you are finished, gently blot your skin with a towel.

Soothing Strategy
Hand Massage

Bring your hands together in front of your chest, palms together. Slowly lower them toward your lap as you continue to press your palms together. You will feel them stretch. Hold for 5 breaths, release, and repeat again holding for 10 breaths.

Extend your right arm at shoulder height, turning your palm away from you and point your fingers straight up as if you were signaling someone to stop. Then, with your left hand, pull the fingers back gently toward your wrist. You will feel the fingers stretch. Hold for 10 breaths and then repeat with your opposite hand.

Extend your arms out in front of you at shoulder height. Spread your fingers as you inhale and make a fist as you exhale. Repeat 5 to 10 times.

Extend your arms out in front of you and make fists with your hands. Next, slowly make circles in the air with your fists, first moving your hands toward each other for 5 circles and then go back the other way. Go slowly and notice how it feels.

With your arms at your sides, simply shake your arms, wrists, and hands for 5 to 10 breaths.

Bend your right elbow in front of your chest and stretch the fingers of your right hand out wide. Grab the web between your thumb and index fingers and massage the skin in that space. Continue for 5 to 10 breaths and then switch to the left hand.

Soothing Strategy
Foot Self-Massage

Begin by sitting upright in a chair. Then, roll your foot over one of the following: a frozen water bottle, a broom handle, or a tennis ball. Or buy a foot roller/massager from a natural health store.

Soothing Strategy
Back Massage (Advanced)

Lay on the floor. Bring your knees up to your chest. Lock your arms around your shins or hold onto the backs of your thighs. Roll gently from one side to the other for 2 minutes. Only try this if you feel comfortable and are flexible enough to get down on the floor. If not, that is okay; skip this and try another exercise.

Massage is the study of anatomy in Braille.
—Jack Meagher

27. Smiling

Smiles have been an integral part of cultures and societies for years, from the Mona Lisa's famous grin to the Buddha's serene smile. Smiling is part of what makes us human, and, of course, we don't need to be the subject of a famous painting or a spiritual guru to practice smiling, either. Think back to the last time you passed someone on the street and that person smiled at you. What did you do in return? If you're like most people, you smiled back. This is an instinctual response, since us humans seem to be wired to mimic others' facial expressions.

Remember the scene in the book and movie *Eat, Pray, Love* when Julia Roberts's guru in Bali teaches her to smile during meditation? "To meditate, only you must smile. Smile with face, smile with mind, and good energy will come to you and clear away dirty energy. Even smile in your liver," said Ketut.

The good news is that, in addition to being polite, smiling can be good for the smiler! Here are just a few of the benefits that result from smiling:

- Reduced stress

- Improved mood

- Lowered blood pressure

- Released endorphins ("feel-good" neurotransmitters)

Interestingly, research supports smiling as a way of coping during a stressful event. In one study, participants who smiled during stressful activities took less time for their heart rates to return to a normal pace when compared with those who didn't smile (Kraft and Pressman 2012). In this study, participants were asked to hold chopsticks in their mouth for a few minutes. Even this manufactured smile helped to reduce heart rates.

Your brain will thank you for smiling instead of frowning, too, since some early research studies have found a correlation between frowning and activation of the *amygdala*—the part of your brain that processes survival emotions like fear. Though scientists have yet to document a direct relationship between frowning and fear, suffice it to say that the relationship appears to exist and supports the importance of smiling. In fact, in another study, participants who had been diagnosed with depression were given Botox injections to prevent frowning. At the conclusion of the study, researchers found that the treatment group felt less depressed than the control group who didn't receive Botox (Finzi and Rosenthal 2014).

Smiling has positive implications for eating as well, because the lower your stress levels and the more relaxed you feel, the less likely you are to find yourself in a situation in which you want to eat for emotional reasons.

Unfortunately, we're not all natural smilers, and as we age, our tendency to smile decreases—considering the fact that children smile an average of 400 times a day, while adults only clock in twenty daily smiles (and for some of us, that number is even lower). However, with practice and conscious awareness, you can start smiling more frequently, enhance your mood, and reduce those negative feelings that lead to emotional eating. So don't reserve your smile for photo-ops anymore; instead, make a point to smile more each day. In fact, continue smiling throughout the day to elevate your mood and maintain a positive frame of mind.

What I like about this technique is that it is completely free, instantaneous, and clinically proven to boost your mood—how can it get better than that? The smiling technique sounds ridiculously simplistic and you may be skeptical. However, I challenge you to give it a try just for one day.

Soothing Strategy
"Duchenne" Smile

The next time a food craving hits, try this smiling exercise, named after the French neuroanatomist Guillaume-Benjamin-Amand Duchenne, who was an early studier of smiles.

First, smile as wide as you can and hold it for 10 seconds. Then try smiling as wide as possible, but this time keep your lips together. Hold for 10 seconds. Repeat each exercise several times. You won't be able to give in to a craving while performing these exercises; plus, that scintillating smile may boost your mood enough to reduce the need to eat!

It's possible to give a polite social smile, but this is not the genuine smile you're aiming for. How can you tell if your smile's the real thing? Real smiles activate both the corners of your mouth *and* the outer corners of your eyes (which is why broad smiles involve crinkling the skin around the outside of your eyes). Smile imposters only curl up the corners of your mouth.

Soothing Strategy
Mirthful Laughter to Calm Down!

Mirthful laughter, or joyous laughter, has many benefits including reducing your cortisol level and blood pressure. In a study on older adults, participants were shown either a distressing video or a comedy video for twenty minutes (Bains et al. 2014). Those who watched the distressing video displayed no changes in their physiology. In contrast, those who watched the comedy had a decrease in blood pressure. A quick and easy smile can be found simply by Googling funny baby videos or comedy videos on YouTube, which has been shown to induce mirthful laughter. Silly babies can keep you in stitches!

Soothing Strategy
Say Cheese, Again!

Practice smiling in a mirror to get used to using the facial muscles that are activated when you grin. If you're having difficulty feeling genuinely happy—or if you feel silly or self-conscious—try to envision a scene or situation that was a happy one for you (such as a recent vacation, getting the promotion at work, or imagining a loved one).

Next, set a smiling goal. How many times each hour or day do you want to smile? Once you set your goal, check in with yourself periodically throughout the day to monitor your progress. If you think you'll forget to keep track, set an alarm on your phone every hour or two as a reminder.

Sometimes your joy is the source of your smile, but sometimes your smile can be the source of your joy. —Thich Nhat Hanh

28. Power Posing

My clients often tell me that they want to have more "control" over their cravings. They feel powerless, like the chocolate is kryptonite. But what if a simple concept like how you stand or control your posture could actually make you a more powerful person in spite of your challenges?

As an adolescent, my friend Alice had to wear a brace to deal with her scoliosis. What she thought was a terrible experience of having to wear a cumbersome contraption during one of her most vulnerable times in life—as a young woman—turned out to be worthwhile in an unexpected way. The brace had straightened her posture for life *and* had inadvertently given her even more power. It's one of the components that made her the person she is today: strong, courageous, and powerful. Interesting research by social psychologist Amy Cuddy and colleagues shows that you can use your body in creative and incredibly simple ways to be more in charge and to feel more confident (Carney, Cuddy, and Yap 2010). Wouldn't that be great when you feel like comfort foods are getting the best of you?

Seems that the concept of *power posing*—standing with force, courage, strength, and character—may produce immediate changes in your body's chemistry. In fact, after just two minutes in a high-power pose—say, hands on hips, legs shoulder width apart, exuding confidence like you were center stage presenting a great idea—the hormone testosterone, a dominance hormone, increases 20 percent, while cortisol, the stress hormone, fades away (Carney, Cuddy, and Yap 2010).

This alpha-stance (think Superman) creates a dominant mindset for which the likes of comfort foods, mindless munching, and soothing yourself with chocolate no longer stand a chance. Why? Because you're the prevailing force, not the food. People who use power pose before a speech or a job interview come into their task more enthusiastic and competent.

Why not use this stance against the chocolate kryptonite? Or, for that matter, any other time a comfort food craving gets the best of you?

Not surprising, the opposite of power posing—standing hunched over, knotted in a ball on the couch, feeling timid in your body stance—affects the opposite of confidence and strength and may lead you to feeling weak, fainthearted, and afraid. These are certainly not the qualities that will help you stand up for yourself against the fridge or any worthy opponent, for that matter. In fact, these postures could have you feeling the opposite, cowering in fear against the cookies in the pantry or that leftover mac and cheese. While of course that's an exaggeration, why not take advantage of every opportunity to feel taller, stand straighter, and exude more strength and power over comfort foods?

Soothing Strategy
Power Pose over Cravings

Be mindful of your body. Notice if you are doing what Amy Cuddy indicates in her research are saboteurs of your power (hunching over, and so on). Try these power poses for 2 minutes. Pick one or try them all.

- Stand like Superwoman. Hands on hips. Chin up.

- Imagine you're the winner of a competition, a medaled Olympiad. Put your arms in the air in the shape of a V (signaling victory!) and hold for 2 minutes.

- Stretch and expand your body, like a chimp in the wild puffing out its chest.

- Cross your arms and roll your shoulders back. Put your chin up.

- Throw your hands in the air. Stand with your feet shoulder width apart. Imagine yourself as a rock performer, your arms wide open, welcoming the applause of your adoring fans.

- Need to avoid the vending machine at work? Place your palms flat on your desk while standing. Lean forward as if you are the boss talking down to your employee sitting in front of you. Say to yourself, "No, you cannot leave your desk to get a candy bar!"

Soothing Strategy
Mindful Standing

Do you hunch over when you are stressed? This can cause further tension and trauma to your body. Try mindful standing:

Imagine the crown of your head is tied to a helium balloon, which is gently pulling you upright.

Stand with your feet apart and your arms hanging by your sides. Feel your body's weight drop down to your feet. Notice any areas that are tense.

Move your arms upward in front of you until they are level with your shoulders. Move them quickly if you need energy or slowly if you need relaxation. Set your arms back down.

Breathe in and out as you do this. Repeat 10 times.

Next, bring your arms out to your sides. Lift until they are out straight (like you are an airplane). Then lower back down. Breathe in and out as you do this. Repeat 10 times.

What you do speaks so loud that I cannot hear what you say.
—Ralph Waldo Emerson

Yoga for Emotional Eating

Maybe you don't practice yoga, you're not into yoga, or you've never even wanted to try yoga. Don't sweat it. But *don't* skip this section. By this point in the book, we are all in agreement that food does calm and soothe us. But there are other things that can calm us, too. Yes, I'm talking about yoga.

I had zero exposure to yoga growing up in northeast Ohio. It wasn't until I was in my late twenties working as a postdoctoral fellow in California when a friend dragged me to a Bikram yoga class (practiced in a *very* warm room). Before I went, I thought, "It probably isn't for me," and figured I wouldn't like it. But the mantra I live by—and I hope you will too—is "You don't know until you try it."

Yoga has now become a staple in my own life as well as in the lives of many of my clients. That being said, I'm not an expert, just an enthusiast. I don't get into complicated poses or twist like a pretzel; I'm still learning, along with everyone else in class. However, I've been practicing long enough to share some helpful and simple yoga tips that practically anyone can do, as well as techniques that my clients tell me work for them.

29. Yoga for Deep Relaxation

As an antianxiety aid and an overall mood lifter, yoga has been found to help those with anxiety and depression better cope. One study showed that after two months of yoga practice, women with anxiety disorders had significantly improved (Javnbakht, Kenari, and Ghasemi 2009). There are many more studies that point to the same conclusion: Yoga is an excellent, natural way to calm and soothe your body.

While yoga is known for its ability to heal everything from a bad back to restoring peace and tranquility, how does this work?

It seems that yoga works on the two nervous systems in the body: sympathetic and parasympathetic. The *sympathetic nervous system*, known as the fight-or-flight response, causes blood pressure to rise, the breath to quicken, and stress hormones like adrenaline and cortisol to flood the body. But today, instead of our system getting triggered by a bear on its hind legs ready to attack, it's being set off by sitting in traffic, a crisis at the office, or dealing with rambunctious kids. Since we never actually fight the bear, all those hormones are stimulating our bodily systems, causing health problems from heart disease to headaches to obesity—because we like to eat to relieve that stress.

Yoga works on the *parasympathetic nervous system* to lower blood pressure and slow the pace of the breath, and to stop the flood of those hormones from ravaging our bodies. Long, slow, deep breathing allows our parasympathetic response to relax and creates healing.

Let's look at some common stressful scenarios. Do any sound familiar to you?

- You are nervously nibbling at your desk as a deadline approaches.

- You find yourself anxious over a confrontation and you are tempted to hide in the kitchen and eat.

- Your stress level is high and all your mind can say is "I need ice cream. Now!"

- You have put the kids to bed and need to unwind, which often means sitting on the couch and mindlessly munching on chips while watching your favorite TV program.

- You are trying to sleep but can't turn your mind off, and you're tempted to get up and get something to eat to help you sleep.

If any of these examples resonate with you, you might be surprised to learn that these—and many more like them—are exactly the types of incidents for which a yoga pose for relaxation may be helpful. Instead of comfort eating, try one of the following yoga poses for five minutes.

Soothing Strategy
Child's Pose

Whenever you're fatigued, need a moment of respite, or simply want to take a time-out, retreat to Child's Pose. It's a resting position that relieves stress and fatigue while stretching the lower back and opening the hips. Here's how you come into the pose:

Come to a kneeling position with your knees a little more than hip-width apart and your toes touching. Then sit back on your heels, keeping your knees apart and your toes touching.

Now bend forward, hinging at your hips, until your chest rests on your thighs and your forehead touches the floor. (*Note:* If your forehead doesn't comfortably reach the floor, place a folded towel or blanket, or even a thick book, beneath it for support.)

Place your arms on the floor alongside your shins, palms facing up. Close your eyes and relax for 5 or more minutes.

Soothing Strategy
Downward-Facing Dog

Downward-Facing Dog is a common yoga pose that reduces fatigue and energizes the body. It provides a deep stretch to hamstrings, shoulders, calves, arches, and hands. Plus, because the heart is higher than the head, it's considered a mild inversion, much like a headstand, and inversions provide benefit for headaches, insomnia, fatigue, and depression. Here's how to get into the pose:

Begin on your hands and knees. Position your wrists directly under your shoulders and your knees directly under your hip bones. Your middle fingers should be pointed straight forward, all fingers spreading wide.

Stretch your arms straight and relax the upper back. Now move your hands 3 inches forward. Distribute weight evenly among the four limbs.

Tuck your toes under and lift your knees off the floor. Your pelvis should reach toward the ceiling while your sit bones point directly behind you. Keep your legs slightly bent. Your body should be in an upside-down V shape.

Press the floor away with your palms as you lift through your pelvis. Lengthen by pointing the sit bones to the ceiling, drawing your shoulder blades into your upper back, and pulling your ribs toward your tailbone. Release your neck muscles, allowing your head to dangle. Try to gently straighten your legs without locking your knees. Aim to get your heels on the floor, though in all likelihood they will remain off the floor, which is fine.

If you can, hold this pose for at least a minute, and aim to build up to 5.

Soothing Strategy
Corpse Pose

Also known as *savasana*, Corpse Pose is a deep-relaxation pose. It can improve memory and concentration, reduce muscle tension, and lower blood pressure and heart rate. It also serves to center and calm the inner mind and restore peace. It's typically practiced at the end of every yoga session. Here's how you get into the pose:

Lie down flat on your back. Place your heels on the floor about hip-width apart, and then allow your feet to gently splay open. Place your arms along your sides with your palms facing up and several inches from your body. Keep your shoulders square. Close your eyes.

Relax your entire body. You may try relaxing one part at a time, if that is easier. Take several belly breaths, as described in chapter 15, Abdominal Breathing.

Continue to lie in Corpse Pose for 5 to 20 minutes. When you are done, slowly roll onto your right side and gently push your way up into a seated position.

Soothing Strategy
Backward Bending

This gentle pose is especially good if you've been sitting at a desk all day, as it helps counteract the bad posture most of us have from being in front of a computer and slouching. Bending backward realigns the spine and relieves stress. It's even helpful for those who suffer from back pain. Here are the steps for a gentle back bend:

Stand up straight with your feet shoulder width apart and your toes turned out slightly.

Place your palms on your lower back just below your waist, with your fingers pointing down.

Moving slowly and gently, bend your head back, then shoulders, and then your back. You may notice your hips moving slightly forward to maintain balance. (*Note:* This should not be a fast-moving or painful pose; if you are feeling discomfort, stop immediately and perhaps try again later, moving more slowly and less forcefully. The smallest movements in this pose are beneficial.) Hold for 5 to 10 seconds—whatever is comfortable. Slowly return to standing. Repeat 10 times.

Yoga teaches us to cure what need not be endured and endure what cannot be cured. —B.K.S. Iyengar

30. Yoga for Sadness and the Blues

Most of us have experienced sadness or depression at some point in our lives. For some, an event like the death of a parent triggers the feelings; for others, there may seem to be no incident in particular that is the cause. But when these feelings start to become chronic—lasting more than a couple weeks and interfering with our work, sleep, and relationships—then our emotional state becomes much more serious and is typically diagnosed as *clinical depression*. A main feature of depression is that there is a lack of energy or desire for what were previously pleasurable activities. The idea of being active at a time when you feel blue may seem counterintuitive, yet this is exactly what is needed to break out of these feelings. While you may not feel like trying yoga when you're down, yoga can be just the thing to help.

The good news is that yoga is a natural way of dealing with the blues, either without medication or as a complement to it. In one study of women with major depressive disorder, participants engaged in an eight-week yoga intervention and were found to have an improvement in symptoms as well as feelings of connectedness to others; they also gained a coping strategy (Kinser et al. 2013).

Researchers are only beginning to understand how a regular yoga practice can help with feelings of sadness and depression.

But a host of theories exists that includes these outcomes: slower breathing, decreased blood pressure, reduction in inflammation, and increased activity along brain pathways to the limbic and cortical areas involved in regulating your mood.

Here are some common scenarios where food is used to help alleviate the blues. Do any of these sound familiar to you?

- Eating comfort food feels like a pick-me-up.

- I find myself overeating when I feel particularly blue.

- I overeat more in the winter when it's overcast and gloomy outside.

- I'm in the dumps about my relationship and find myself looking for food that will make me feel better.

- I just can't seem to shake this dark cloud hanging over me. Eating temporarily fills the void even though the feelings resurface later.

If any of these examples resonate with you, yoga can help. The following yoga moves are known to help relieve feelings of sadness, gloominess, and depression. Try them by themselves anytime or as a complement to a regimen you already have in place to combat depression.

Soothing Strategy
Sun Breath

This movement will help you feel more energetic and optimistic. Traditionalists face east when doing sun breaths to symbolize the spiritual dawn of awareness. Try it first thing in the morning.

Stand upright with your feet hip-width apart and your arms at your sides. Exhale completely.

As you inhale, raise your arms out to the sides and above your head. Extend your fingers upward and feel a stretch along your sides. Look up at your hands if that feels okay. Press your palms together overhead, but only if you can do so without discomfort. Hold your breath slightly.

As you exhale, slowly circle your arms back down to your sides. This is one Sun Breath.

Repeat 6 to 8 times.

Soothing Strategy
Forward Fold

The simple act of bending forward creates length and space in the spine, strengthens the thighs and knees, and relieves tension. It also can help reduce stress, anxiety, depression, and fatigue—which you may have been trying to treat with comfort eating. Here's how you get into this pose:

Stand upright with your feet hip-width apart and your arms at your sides. Keep a slight bend in your knees. Inhale completely.

As you exhale, slowly hinge at your hips, lowering your torso forward. Your arms should hang down in front of you with fingertips skimming the floor. If you can't touch the floor, simply hang your hands as low as they go, rest fingertips on your shins, or place your fingertips on blocks for support. Let your head hang. Release all tension in your shoulders and neck. Keep your legs bent if your hamstrings are tight; straighten your legs for a deeper stretch.

Breathe deeply. Hold the pose for 30 seconds to 1 minute. This is one Forward Fold.

To come up to standing, bend your knees slightly and roll up one vertebrae at a time. Repeat the sequence 6 to 8 times.

Soothing Strategy
Cobra Pose

Like the other poses in this chapter, this yoga posture helps reduce anxiety, stress, and depression. It increases blood and oxygen flow, which is invigorating and can help elevate your mood. Here's how you get into the pose:

Begin lying facedown on a flat, firm surface. Your feet should be hip-width apart, and the tops of your feet should rest flat on the floor—do not tuck the toes under.

Place your hands under your shoulders with fingers pointing forward. Hug your elbows in tight against your sides. Inhale while pressing through the tops of your feet, pelvis, and hands. Gently lift your head and chest off the floor, keeping your lower ribs on the floor.

Draw your shoulder blades down away from your ears and flat against your back. Slightly straighten your arms; there should still be a generous bend at your elbows. Keep your gaze toward the floor, especially if you have neck pain. Feel a gentle stretch in the back.

Hold for 30 seconds to 1 minute. Release by exhaling slowly and lowering your chest and forehead back to the floor. Place your arms back at your sides. This is one Cobra Pose. Repeat the pose 6 times.

Soothing Strategy
Half Sun Salutation

Even one round of Half Sun Salutation can make a huge difference in the way you feel. It can go a long way to lifting sadness and depression. Practicing several rounds (10 to 20) will have a dramatic effect on your moods. Try it in the morning or anytime you feel particularly blue.

Stand upright with your feet hip-width apart and your arms at your sides. Exhale completely.

As you inhale, do one Sun Breath. But when you circle your arms back down on the exhale, continue straight into Forward Fold.

Once you are folded forward, on an inhale, press your fingers into your shins, arms straight, and stretch your upper body forward with a flat back. Use the next exhale to return to Forward Fold.

Use the next inhale to smoothly move back to standing and through another Sun Breath. On the next exhale, return to standing with your arms at your sides. This is one Half Sun Salutation. Use one breath per movement, and repeat 6 to 8 times or more.

The yoga mat is a good place to turn when talk therapy and antidepressants aren't enough. —Amy Weintraub

31. Yoga for Work Stress

If you didn't know that you could decompress from the stress of work with yoga, you don't know what you've been missing. Yoga can help with specific problems in your life, and many moves have been adapted to perform in a chair. You can practice these easy and simple chair moves right at your desk!

Many of my clients report that the majority of their stress eating happens at work. It makes sense. You might spend eight, nine, twelve hours—the majority of your day—at work or school. Job and work stress, no matter where your position falls on the work hierarchy, can eat away at you. Bosses, long hours, difficult commutes, coworker conflicts, and challenging customers are all a recipe for stress.

A study in the *American Journal of Clinical Nutrition* found that job burnout is highly associated with emotional eating (Nevanperä et al. 2012). The study looked at 230 working women who said they were burned out and highly stressed, and therefore were emotional eaters. Researchers concluded that the way to halt emotional eating is not to clear the pantry of junk food but to clear the mind and body of stress. It seems that addressing the stress is how you curb comfort eating.

Many of my clients report that they can't even leave their desk, classroom, or cubicle. Therefore, I'm including some simple yoga exercises you can do right in your office—right in your chair, in fact—that will give you the same benefits that you would achieve if you were in a yoga studio: relaxation, decompression, and reduced stress.

Here are some common situations when food is used to help alleviate work stress. Do any of these sound familiar to you?

- You are under pressure to meet a deadline and all you can think about is food.

- You get nervous about Monday-morning team meetings and find yourself unable to avoid the muffins and donuts.

- You can't stand your coworker. Whenever she walks by you feel like hiding.

- You find yourself hungry when you arrive at your stressful job even though you already ate breakfast at home.

- Your boss is impossible to please so you're always on the defensive.

If any of these examples resonate with you, then I have a great solution. The following chair exercises adapted from yoga can help to alleviate work stress, prevent burnout, and induce relaxation—and thereby lessen your cravings and emotional eating habits.

Soothing Strategy
Chair Pose

Sit in a chair with your spine straight and feet firmly on the floor. On an inhalation, raise your arms toward the ceiling.

Reach hands straight up above your head while letting your shoulder blades slide down your back. Lengthen your back and sides. Pull your navel in toward your spine. Feel the stretch. Pause for a few seconds and lower hands on an exhale.

Repeat 5 times.

Soothing Strategy
Towel Stretch

Sit in a chair with your spine straight and feet firmly on the floor. With your palms facing down, hold the ends of a towel or rope taut in front of you. Place your hands wide apart.

Lift the towel slowly over your head, pulling the ends of the towel outward. Pause. Then move your arms behind you. You might feel your hands shift along the towel, which is fine. You should feel a stretch in the front of your shoulders. If you feel any discomfort, try placing your hands farther apart on the towel.

Now slowly bring your arms back up over your head and to your front. Repeat this sequence 5 times.

Soothing Strategy
Cat-Cow Stretch

Sit upright in a chair with your spine straight and both feet firmly on the floor. Rest your hands on your knees or thighs.

On an inhale, move your chest upward and forward, and drop your shoulders back and down so the shoulder blades lie are flat against your back. You should feel a gentle arch in the upper back. This is a modified Cow Pose.

On the exhale, round your spine, pulling your navel in and letting your shoulders and head drop forward. This is a modified Cat Pose.

Repeat this cycle, moving into Cow Pose on the inhalation and into Cat Pose on the exhalation, for 5 breaths.

Soothing Strategy
Forward Chair Bend

Sit upright in a chair with your spine straight and your feet firmly on the floor. With a deep inhalation through the nose, raise your arms straight above your head. Stretch your fingers toward the ceiling and feel a stretch along your sides.

On the exhalation, hinge at your hips, slowly bending forward over your thighs. Rest your chest on your thighs and extend your arms straight alongside your ears and toward the wall in front of you. Your back and arms should feel flat like a tabletop. Then slowly lower your arms, ultimately resting your hands on the floor, if they reach. Allow your head to hang freely.

On the next inhalation, slowly lift upward, keeping your back and arms straight and in one line, raising chest off knees, until you are sitting upright again with arms straight overhead and hands reaching for the ceiling.

Repeat 5 times.

Soothing Strategy
Chair Warrior

Sit upright in a chair with your spine straight and your feet firmly on the floor. Now shift your hips so that your torso is facing the wall on your right. Move your right leg so that the knee is also facing the wall on your right. Place your right foot flat on the floor with toes also facing the wall on your right.

Now stretch your left leg straight behind you. With the left toes on the floor, and your heel raised, stretch your heel toward the left wall. You may need to sit closer to the edge of your seat to get into this pose.

Keep your torso facing the right wall. As you inhale, raise your arms up to the ceiling. Keep your shoulders down and your shoulder blades flat against your back while you stretch your fingers toward the ceiling. You should feel a gentle stretch along your arms, chest, groin, and legs.

Hold for 5 breaths. Repeat on the other side.

Soothing Strategy
Hamstring Stretch

Stand about an arm's-length distance from your chair and face it.

Place your right heel on the seat of your chair. A slight bend in your right knee is okay, but work toward straightening it, if that feels comfortable. Your standing left leg should be straight, and your left toes should be facing forward. It's a common mistake to turn the toes outward, which is bad form. For the best stretch, keep the entire body—both sets of toes, your hips, and your torso—facing forward.

Flex your right foot and slowly hinge at the hips, folding forward, keeping your back straight. Come forward only as far as feels comfortable without bending your right leg or rounding your back. You should feel a stretch in your hamstrings and back.

Hold for 5 deep breaths, then repeat on the other side. Repeat the sequence 5 times.

Yoga is not about touching your toes, it is what you learn on the way down. —Jigar Gor

32. Yoga for Anger

Anger is your body's way of letting you know that your boundaries have been crossed. Sometimes this anger is expressed in healthy ways, and other times in unhealthy ways—like when it urges you to emotionally eat. Some people literally stuff their feelings with food.

If anger is repressed with food, you may miss the important message it has for you. That message might be as small as "You are angry," in which case all you need do is acknowledge this and move on. Or it might be as big as, "You hate your job and need to do something proactive about it." Or you may have unresolved feelings about something, in which case you should probably explore them.

It's very important to deal with anger. Avoiding it—or stuffing it with food—won't make it go away. Looking at it and feeling it, although seemingly counterintuitive for an emotion that brings discomfort, can offer the opportunity to stop emotional eating. It's not easy! Particularly for women, who may not have been taught what to do with anger besides hide it away.

Did you know that a regular yoga practice can help release those angry feelings? Yoga not only helps you home in on your anger and figure out why you're angry; it can help you set an intention to release that anger as well as help you resolve it.

One small study took a group of twenty-six women and divided them into different stress-management programs to deal with anger (Granath et al. 2006). One was cognitive therapy and the other was yoga. At the end of four months there were few differences between the two groups, emphasizing that both cognitive therapy and a practice of yoga were equally beneficial when it came to managing stress.

What's more, specific studies on yoga's effects on anger are beginning to show promising results. One such study on the psychological health of older adults found that yoga participants showed greater improvements in anger levels than those who were assigned to a different exercise group (Bonura and Tenenbaum 2014).

This may be promising news for preventing heart attacks and stroke in people prone to angry responses and for helping those cope with and release pent-up anger.

Here are some common examples of times when food is used to help alleviate anger. Do any of these sound familiar to you?

- You say to yourself, "I just don't care what I eat."

- You say to yourself, "What the hell? What I eat doesn't matter anyway."

- You get angry at a family member or friend for seemingly being able to eat anything.

- You hate your body and it makes you very upset.

- You feel angry but don't dare say anything, so you eat something that you think will make you feel better.

If any of these examples resonate with you, then look no further. The following yoga exercises can help you manage your anger so that you don't resort to emotional eating. Keep in mind that a combination of breathing exercises, physical exercises, and meditation practiced together will yield the best results for most people. If your anger continues to rage out of control, seek a psychotherapist, who can provide you with additional coping tools. Remember: It's not about bottling up, ignoring, or stuffing down your anger with food. Many of my clients talk about turning their anger against themselves. They hear themselves say angry statements like "To heck with it, I don't care what I eat" or "I am a failure. I might as well eat the entire thing." Use the techniques in this section to tone down anger and ride through it skillfully, without throwing fuel on your feelings.

Soothing Strategy
Engaging the Mula Bandha

It's thought that anger, along with other intense emotions, is held in the abdomen. By engaging the muscles of the pelvic floor (*mula bandha*), this exercise channels your anger, allowing its energy to expand throughout the entire body. Here's how to do it:

First, reread the directions for Skull-Shining Breath, in chapter 18.

Next, lie on your back on a flat, firm surface. Bend your legs and place your feet flat on the ground and hip-width apart. Stretch your arms close to your sides, palms facing down.

Engage your stomach muscles by pulling the navel toward the spine. Feel that your core muscles are engaged. Now raise your feet, knees still bent, to a height that challenges your muscles but that you can sustain for at least 1 minute. You might raise your knees so they are directly over your hips with your shins parallel to the ground (easiest), you might raise your feet only a few inches off the ground (challenging), or you might even straighten your legs (hardest).

Take a deep inhale, and on an exhale begin Skull-Shining Breath. Practice for 1 to 1.5 minutes. Repeat up to 3 times, if that's available to you.

Soothing Strategy
Seated Half Twist

Twists balance the spine, expand the chest, and increase the flow of blood throughout the body. Moreover, they massage our internal organs, cleansing them of toxins and loosening tension. Think of twisting as wringing out your anger!

Sit upright on a flat, firm surface up with your legs stretched out straight in front of you.

Bend the left leg and place the heel of the left foot beside the right hip, close to the groin. Allow the left thigh and knee to rest on the floor.

Next, place your right foot flat on the floor outside of your left thigh. Your right knee should be facing the ceiling.

On a deep inhale, raise your arms above your head and stretch your fingers toward the ceiling. On an exhale, turn your torso slightly to the right and slower lower your arms. Place your left palm on the outside of your right knee and your right hand behind you. Either your right fingertips or your whole palm should be on the floor.

With every inhale, expand your chest and grow taller. With every exhale, gently twist from the waist, shoulders, and neck—in that order. Keep your spine elongated. Take long deep breaths for 1 minute.

To come out of the pose, gently release the twist and face forward again. Bring both legs straight in front of you. Then repeat on the other side.

Soothing Strategy
Seated Forward Fold

This yoga pose is a variation of one in chapter 30. It is good for releasing tension in the back, shoulders, and neck and for increasing the flow of positive energy. You can practice this pose on its own, or, for a longer sequence, start with a few minutes of Cooling Breath (chapter 19) and end with 5 minutes in Corpse Pose (chapter 29).

Sit upright on a flat firm surface with your legs stretched out straight in front of you. Keep your legs together or hip-width apart. Flex your feet and keep your spine elongated.

On a deep inhale, raise both arms above your head and stretch fingers toward the ceiling.

On an exhale, slowly hinge at your hips, bending forward, arms still in line with your spine. As you move toward your legs, imagine your sternum reaching for your toes, rather than your forehead to your knees. The idea is to keep your back straight and reach forward. Move slowly. Only bend so far that you can maintain a straight back. Hold this position and breathe for 20 to 40 seconds.

Then gently round your spine and lower your arms to your legs. If your head can rest on your knees, allow it to do so; otherwise, simply let go of the upper body and allow the head, neck, shoulders, back, and arms to relax and hang. Hold for at least 1 minute or as long as you like.

It's your body. Tell it what to do. —Chris Powell

33. Yoga for Energy

Sure, you can take up yoga to calm yourself, get toned, lift depression, reduce stress, burn calories, and reduce your cravings. But are you aware that a regular yoga practice builds energy? Yoga increases blood flow and levels of hemoglobin and red blood cells, which allows more oxygen to reach the body's cells, enhancing all their functions.

Often my clients tell me that yoga both tires and energizes them, which sounds like a huge contradiction. However, take one or two yoga sessions and you'll soon understand. While yoga is exercise, and exercise is fatiguing, the combination of stretching, movement, and breath serves to increase your energy overall. Yoga builds energy by adjusting hormone levels and by specifically reducing cortisol. Some yoga poses reduce fatigue while those that force you to balance improve your focus, attention, and concentration.

How does yoga give you energy and help fight comfort eating? We tend to eat unnecessarily when we are bored and tired, because eating stimulates our senses and can give a short boost of energy. The reasoning is that if you aren't bored or tired, you probably will eat less.

Here are some situations in which boredom eating typically happens. Do any of these scenarios sound familiar to you?

- You drink a lot of coffee because you constantly feel exhausted.

- You tend to eat something "to keep you going" midday.

- You find that you're always hungry.

- You feel like you're dragging yourself around.

- Even when you do get sleep, it never feels like enough.

- You find yourself reaching for carbs, which give you an immediate rush of energy, but then your energy levels crash later.

If you can relate to any of these scenarios, then try the following poses. You should feel a noticeable improvement in your energy level.

Soothing Strategy
The Conductor

This exercise helps you to awaken and cleanse the body and mind. It requires you to separate your breath into three parts as you inhale while doing a slightly modified Sun Breath (see chapter 30, Yoga for Sadness and the Blues). This "salute to the sun" is said to get your blood pumping, increase circulation, and raise the heart rate. Because of this, you are awakened with new energy. It is easier than it sounds!

Stand upright with your feet hip-width apart, toes facing forward, arms at your side. Exhale completely. Inhale one-third of a full breath as you take your arms to shoulder height in front of you. Pause.

Now, continue to inhale another third of the way as you take your arms out to the sides at shoulder height. Pause. Then inhale the final third of your breath as you take your arms straight up overhead. Pause.

Exhale loudly through your mouth, as if you are noisily trying to fog a pane of glass in front of your mouth, while you hinge from your hips, letting your arms circle down and your torso fold forward. You may keep your knees bent if that feels more comfortable. Release the muscles in your neck, allowing your head to hang loose. Allow your hands to do the same; they do not have to touch the floor. Exhale completely. This is 1 round of the Conductor exercise.

On a one-third inhalation, return to the first standing pose with your arms out in front of you and continue the movement, repeating 6 to 8 times.

Soothing Strategy
Mountain Pose

This basic standing pose is the backbone of other standing poses and is thought to allow the internal organs to function optimally, improving respiration, digestion, and circulation and making you feel more energetic and alive.

Stand upright, feet flat on the ground, big toes touching, heels slightly apart. Balance weight evenly throughout the feet. Tighten your thigh muscles and lengthen your tailbone toward the floor. Press your navel toward your spine. Imagine a line of energy from your feet to your inner thighs to your pelvis and then through your torso, neck, and head.

Release your shoulders down, pressing your shoulder blades flat against your back. Allow your arms to hang at your sides, palms facing out, fingers splayed. Engage your triceps and biceps as you lengthen your arms. Center your head directly over your pelvis, chin parallel to the floor. Keep your mouth neutral, tongue relaxed, eyes soft. Hold this pose for 30 seconds to a minute while breathing deeply. *Note:* If you feel any lower back pain, move your feet hip-distance apart.

Soothing Strategy
Legs up the Wall Pose

Often done at the end of a yoga practice before Corpse Pose (see chapter 29, Yoga for Deep Relaxation), Legs up the Wall Pose is a rejuvenating inverted pose for all levels of yogis. It provides relief to the legs, feet, spine, and nervous system and is both deeply relaxing as well as energizing. Because you are mildly inverted, you receive benefits such as reduced headaches, fatigue, depression, and insomnia.

Place a firm pillow or bolster against a wall. Sit with your left side up against the wall, your lower back against the pillow. Turn slowly to the left, bringing your legs up onto the wall, scooting your lower back onto the pillow as you lower your mid- and upper back to the floor. Your shoulders and head should rest comfortably on the floor.

Scoot your behind close to the wall and keep your arms extended and slightly out from your sides, palms facing up. Your lower back should be fully supported by the pillow. Release any tension where your thigh bones meet at your hip socket. Your legs should be straight (or with a slight bend), feet hip-width apart.

Close your eyes. Relax in this position for 5 to 10 minutes, breathing with awareness.

To come out of the pose, bend at the knees and slowly slide your legs down to the floor, turning your torso on its side as you do. Use your hands to push yourself up into a seated position.

The energy of the mind is the essence of life. —Aristotle

Expressive Arts Therapy

Sometimes words aren't enough. We think about our problems over and over, then talk to our friends about them, but nothing changes. Enter the expressive arts, which are also sometimes known as "creative arts therapies." The expressive arts—such as music therapy, writing therapy, dance therapy, and art therapy—help to bypass your everyday thinking and take you to a deeper inner place, where you can tap in to the creative process to positively effect change.

But make no mistake, the art therapies are not about making pretty pictures, beautiful music, or crafting the perfect poem. They are solely about healing and therefore can be used by anyone—creative arts training or not. As you will see, you don't have to be a musician to use music therapy, or a dancer to use dance therapy. All you need is a willingness and openness to engage in the process!

34. Writing Therapy

Writing is something that we all know how to do and often take for granted. But did you know that writing can be very therapeutic? Best of all, you only need a pen and paper! With a little focus and direction, writing can become a powerful tool for personal growth, change, and managing cravings. Writing eases difficult feelings and gives you a place to record them. In psychology, we call this a "container." You get to see patterns in your behavior, thinking, and emotions, and you start to understand the cause and effect of themes in your life.

There are many kinds of writing therapies. Journaling is probably the most common and least structured, as you can record whatever you like: daily reflections, wishes for the future, commentary about your life, secrets, dreams, a record of your emotions—virtually anything that comes to mind. Memoirs and autobiographies are a longer, more formal kinds of writing that can be tremendously healing and cathartic. Other forms of therapeutic writing include poetry and structured writing exercises. What's more, sharing your writing with others can be very healing, as it allows you to connect to others and to your humanity. If you have any interest in exploring therapeutic writing, I highly encourage you to pursue it.

Writing therapy doesn't have to take a lot of time or be as long as a dissertation. Even one or two words jotted down on a calendar or in a pocket-size notebook can help. Your writing doesn't even have to be full sentences or make sense to anyone else but you. Spelling and punctuation don't count, and no one but you will read your work (unless, of course, you decide to share).

I particularly urge people to write while the emotions are happening, while they are still "hot." Emotions change over time, so it's beneficial to capture those feelings as they're coming to you. Those who bring in their journals to counseling are able to give a candid account of how they were feeling, not the remembered and revised version.

The best benefit of journaling? Writing down your feelings helps you to connect the dots between events in your life. This is important for getting in charge of cravings and emotional eating. Triggers for emotional eating don't always happen a few seconds before you eat the cookie. Sometimes it is an event that began two days before. For example, Janice, my client, noticed she had about a twenty-four-hour delay between things that bothered her (conflict with her boyfriend) and emotional eating (sugary snacks and carbs). It wasn't easy to make that connection without the aid of a journal. Now that she knows about the time lag, she's able to prepare ahead of time for when she suspects she'll be vulnerable to emotional eating.

A regular practice of writing has been shown to provide a host of health benefits including stress reduction, lower blood pressure, increased feelings of well-being, improved memory, improved mood, enhanced self-esteem, and weight loss. A study reported in *Psychological Science* (Logel and Cohen 2012) showed that women who wrote in a journal about their most important values were able to lose weight (on average 3.4 pounds) versus women who wrote about less-important issues, who actually gained weight (on average 2.8 pounds). The researchers theorize that writing about things that matter improved participants' self-esteem and self-resolve. This makes sense. When you are writing and thinking about what truly matters in the grand scheme of your life, whether you eat a doughnut or not seems to feel less important. You reaffirm what matters.

Soothing Strategy
Giving Voice

Grab your journal and a pen, and stand in the center of a room. Take a moment to think of a strong emotion or craving.

Give that emotion or craving a name (for example, "insecurity," "fear," or "candy").

Walk to a part of the room where you would most like to put that feeling or craving.

Begin to write in your journal as if the emotion or craving is speaking. Use these prompts to help:

I am _____ [name the feeling or craving].

I want _____ .

I feel _____ .

I wish _____ .

Notice how you feel. Write down any other thoughts or feelings that you might be experiencing.

Soothing Strategy
Poetry Therapy

Think of a word that represents a strong emotion or craving that you are having. Pull out your journal and write that word vertically on the page. For example, if I choose the emotion anxiety, I would write it like this:

A

N

X

I

E

T

Y

Now you are going to create a poem by using each letter to start a phrase. For example…

Am angry at my mother.

Nothing I eat will make it better.

…and so on.

Alternatively, write your word vertically in the far right margin of the page. Then begin a phrase starting at the left margin and ending with a word that begins with the letter listed on that particular line. For example…

I think I'm craving an Apple.

I have trouble sleeping at Night.

…and so on.

Be honest and get creative. It can be a lot of fun. Your poem can be created just about anywhere, at any time, and you will be surprised at how therapeutic it is.

Soothing Strategy
Gratitude Journal

If standard journaling feels too overwhelming or you think you don't have time for it, try a simple gratitude journal. Dedicate a notebook specifically to writing down three to five things that you are grateful for every day. Try to come up with new items every day. Don't ignore the journal if you've had a bad day; instead, challenge yourself to find the positive in any negative situation. In doing so, you will change your outlook on your situation and perhaps become more optimistic in general. In fact, you might find that you are more relaxed and sleeping more soundly too (Wood et al. 2009)!

Here are some helpful prompts:

Today, the person I am grateful for is:

Today, the activity I am grateful for is:

Today, the food I am grateful for is:

In times of stress, the best thing we can do for each other is to listen with our ears and our hearts and to be assured that our questions are just as important as our answers.
—Fred "Mister" Rogers

35. Music Therapy

Let me say this right upfront: When it comes to singing or playing a musical instrument it's best I do it alone, like in the car or while showering. But not having any musical talent doesn't stop me for a minute. I love music and the therapeutic effects it has! The good news is that you don't have to be a virtuoso or have perfect pitch to benefit from music therapy. As you'll discover in the music therapy exercises that follow, there are a variety of easy ways to use and incorporate music into your life. Of course, if you already have the capacity to sing or play an instrument, even better, since you can learn to use those skills to combat comforting eating.

My clients talk about music all the time. When they hear a song that perfectly articulates how they're feeling, they tell me about it. If I haven't heard the song, I write it down and play it later because it gives me deep insight into what my client is feeling and why this particular song is having an impact. Hearing their song gives us more information to work with. It doesn't surprise me that emotional eaters are drawn to music therapy. They are often people who experience feelings profoundly and therefore seem to experience music on a deeper level.

Music is incredibly soothing. Why? Well, we're hardwired for sound and vibrations, for one. When words cannot communicate a thought or feeling for one reason or another, music can reach us at deep levels of our being. We can then face things we're feeling and perhaps express ourselves more easily. Just think about your favorite song from high school or one that is associated with your first romantic partner; most likely a host of feelings and images come to mind. What about songs associated with religious practices or ceremonies? Does Christmas music or *The Star-Spangled Banner* evoke a feeling of nostalgia or patriotism?

Even more interesting, music alleviates stress. In a study of sixty healthy women who either listened to music, listened to the sound of rippling water, or rested in silence before a stressor was introduced, researchers found that the music group experienced the most stress relief (Thoma et al. 2013). Researchers concluded that listening to music before experiencing stress helped the women recover faster. Music therapy is used for a wide variety of applications both by clinicians (music therapists) and by individuals who want effective ways to deal with stressors and the challenges of everyday living.

Music encourages brain waves to resonate in sync with the beat; faster beats improve concentration and alertness while slower beats produce a calming, meditative state. Most of us have had the experience of hearing a piece of music that has raised our energy level or relaxed us. Along with the mind-body changes come measurable changes in breathing and heart rate. Music also encourages optimism and stimulates creativity. And, yes, studies have also proven that music impacts how you eat.

Interestingly, music can even change your perception of taste. In one study participants listened to various music genres—hip-hop, rock, classical, and jazz—while they ate both emotional and nonemotional foods (chocolate milk and bell peppers, respectively). Researchers found that music genre can alter both the flavor pleasantness and overall impression of foods eaten (Fiegel et al. 2014). And the speed of the music makes a difference as well. The slower the music, the less people ate (Wansink and van Ittersum 2012). Diners who ate with soft lighting and music reported enjoying their meal more than those who ate in the typical fast food setting.

The theory is that in a more relaxed dining environment people eat slower. This allows them to feel full sooner and prevents overeating. When you eat fast, as people who ate with bright lights and loud, fast music in the background did, you tend to wolf down your food so you can get out of the situation faster. Since your body doesn't register fullness as quickly, you tend to overeat.

Soothing Strategy
Pick a Song

If particularly strong feelings come up after this exercise, consider writing about them or discussing them with a trusted friend or counselor.

Pick a song that represents a strong emotion or craving that you are experiencing. Play the song, listening carefully to words, the music, and your feelings.

Once the song is over, notice how you feel. Has the craving or emotion changed in some way?

Now pick another song that gently helps to transition you to a more balanced emotional state.

Soothing Strategy
Play Any Instrument

Pick an instrument, any instrument. A tambourine, small drum, slide flute, or kazoo will do just fine. If you have the ability to play a more complex instrument, then you can certainly do so! Instruments like flutes can change your breathing pattern, which can help you calm down. Hitting a drum can alter your heartbeat. Playing any instrument is a simple distraction from whatever is stewing on your mind.

Grab an instrument. Close your eyes, take a few deep breaths, and get in touch with strong feelings or cravings.

Begin to use the instrument in a way that reflects your emotion or craving. Continue to play until it naturally feels like it's time to stop.

Notice how you feel. Has the emotion or craving changed? Are there new emotions?

Soothing Strategy
Your Story in Song

Think back to when you had your first emotional food craving. As you reflect on this time, notice the phases in your life that you pass as you arrive at your earliest memory of an emotional craving. Give a name to each phase, such as "occasionally," "living in the country," "intense cravings," "relationship problems," "five years ago." Go for 5 to 10 phases, if possible, but fewer is okay.

Now find a song or piece of music that represents each phase. If possible, put all of them together in chronological order on a disc or digital file.

Play the songs and listen to the words and music. Pay attention to any feelings that rise.

When done, notice how you feel. What has changed? You may want to journal about any strong feelings.

Take a music bath once or twice a week for a few seasons.
You will find it is to the soul what a water bath is to the body.
—Oliver Wendell Holmes

36. Dance Therapy

Throughout time various cultures and religions have used dance to express emotions, tell stories, treat illness, celebrate, foster communal ties, and connect with their spirituality. As is with most of the modalities in this book, dance therapy is a mind-body approach that enters the realm of healing through movement in the body. Dance therapists view movement of the body as another means for expressing the psyche and for communicating through the metaphor of movement. Dance therapy can be done in groups or through an individual practice and is often used to treat social, emotional, cognitive, and physical issues.

One of the unique benefits of dance therapy is that it encourages you to take charge of your body, connect with yourself at a deeper level, and safely become more aware of your emotions and internal sensations. This is particularly helpful for people who have eating issues, as they often have had some kind of trauma that has caused them to become disconnected from their body and feelings. On a clinical level, research has shown that dance therapy helps improve body image, reduces depression and moodiness, improves self-esteem, and reduces stress. These are also important factors influencing weight loss and managing cravings.

Additionally, dance therapy offers many of the benefits of exercise: improved flexibility, enhanced coordination, better balance, a release of tension in the body, improved circulation, healthier muscle tone, and a greater sense of well-being (Strassel et al. 2011). In a study on forty adolescents (mean age sixteen) with mild depression, the impact of dance therapy was put to the test. For twelve weeks, participants either took part in dance therapy or a control group (Jeong et al. 2005). At the end of the study, plasma serotonin concentration increased and dopamine concentration decreased in the dance therapy group (versus placebo).

At the end of the day, whether you are feeling chronically blue or just need to feel better fast, dancing can help change your neurobiology. As one of my favorite clients likes to say, "Dance it out!"

Soothing Strategy
Let's Get Positive

Be sure to have a clear space where you can comfortably move. You can practice when you experience an urge to snack or any other time.

Turn on some music of your choosing. Instead of giving in to a craving or strong emotion, come up with a positive statement. For example, if you are feeling the urge to eat for stress-related reasons, what is something positive you can say to yourself? How about something like, "We all experience stress; there are many healthy ways to deal with it."

As you start to repeat your positive statement over and over again, create a small movement with your body that represents or accentuates this. Maybe sway your arms or hips or move from side to side in a slow, wavy motion.

For 5 minutes, continue to repeat the statement and movement.

Notice how you feel. What has changed?

Soothing Strategy
Moving from the Inside Out

This exercise is deceptively simple but can be very powerful. Here also, be sure to practice where you can comfortably move.

Turn on your favorite music. Stand in the center of an unobstructed space and close your eyes. Turn your awareness inside and notice any feelings, sensations, or emotions.

Select one of those feelings, sensations, or emotions and let that begin to move you in some way. Just allow it to guide you, rather than you guiding it.

Continue to move until you feel complete with the exercise. When done, notice how you feel.

Dance first. Think later. It's the natural order.
—Samuel Beckett

37. Art Therapy

On many occasions, my clients bring in crafts, drawings, sculptures, collages, or paintings (or cell phone snapshots of them) that they've made between sessions. Seeing their art is extremely helpful during counseling. Art often communicates something about how my clients are feeling in a totally nonverbal way; I can look at their creations and understand more about them. And you don't have to be an art major or Picasso to make art or receive its benefits.

Let's face it: sometimes it's *hard* to put how you're feeling into words. In fact, this is a significant struggle for people who have elements of what is known as *alexithymia*, or difficulty putting feelings into words, and who overeat. Alexithymia is an inability to recognize one's emotions and their subtleties, and to explain them. Creating art is less daunting than giving a coherent, dissertation-like thesis of what you are feeling inside. Instead, making art gives an opportunity for an enriching and pleasurable experience of introspection.

You might be surprised to learn what your art says about you. After all, isn't that why we visit art galleries and admire artists—to be inspired, to understand something that we didn't understand before we viewed the art, and to get into the soul of the artist and comprehend what he meant to share?

Art also taps in to the right brain, which has been shown to enhance problem solving, improve leadership, and foster innovative thinking. Harvard medical students are taking art-appreciation courses, because analyzing paintings was shown to help future doctors assess patients' symptoms (Naghshineh et al. 2008). And corporations bring in artists and provide art classes to help their managers access their creative right brain.

One of my clients told me about the power of art in her life. She said it worked so well that it was like flipping the off switch on her emotional eating. She used to munch nervously while on stressful phone calls. Then one day she began doodling on a small pad of paper near her phone. Not only did the time fly by, she didn't eat a single bite! During each call from that day forward, she let her pen fly around the paper while she listened. She reduced her stress and eliminated snacking.

Can creating art really help when you are totally stressed out? Art has been shown to improve moods even for those who are experiencing a stress level that's off the charts. A case in point are recent studies on art therapy with various groups of people experiencing high levels of stress: patients with breast cancer, prisoners, people who've experienced trauma, those with traumatic brain injuries, and more (Slayton, D'Archer, and Kaplan 2010). This review of studies pointed to several mood benefits with short art interventions. So if creating art is helpful for people in extremely stressful situations, it's likely to work for the more mundane types of everyday stress that lead you to comfort eat. Even if a paintbrush has intimidated you in the past or you've said, "I can't draw, paint, or sculpt!" give it a shot. You might be surprised.

Soothing Strategy
Try Zentangle

This is one of my favorite art strategies. When you have the urge to emotionally eat, try Zentangle, created by Rick and Maria Thomas. The objective is to create a beautiful design from repeated patterns. It's a fun, relaxing, and lighthearted activity that doesn't cost a cent; it's also portable and doesn't require technical skills to be creative. My clients have told me that it's soothing, as it almost puts them into a trancelike state. It's a form of mindfulness, and because you need to focus all of your attention on the present moment without judgment, it makes the experience like a meditation too.

Zentangle relies on your intuition, allowing your subconscious to take you wherever you want to go. There is no right or wrong way to do it. It's a nonverbal method of journaling that results in stress relief, improved coordination, and focus. It's also a great metaphor for life. You can't erase ink, so you have to work any "mistakes" you make into the pattern. In other words, nothing in life is perfect—the key is to accept this and adjust to it. Also, Zentangle doesn't elicit criticism since there is no exact way to do it.

Get a sheet of heavy card stock and a black pen or Sharpie. (The traditional way to do Zentangle is to use graph paper; the squares can help you to create a repeated pattern of shapes.) Now draw. It can be whatever you want: small squares, lines, designs, hearts, common shapes, repeated symbols, and so on. They can be drawn vertically, horizontally, overlapping—however you like. It's as simple as that. (See http://www.zentangle.com for ideas.)

Don't rush, judge, or feel pressured to do anything in particular. Let your pen move where it wishes. Follow along. Be in the moment!

Soothing Strategy
Food Portrait

Get out a piece of paper and something to draw with. Now illustrate how your craving for food looks right now. Maybe the craving feels all encompassing and you draw yourself in the middle of a big ball. Or maybe it feels like a ball and chain hanging from your neck or ankle, and so you draw that. Whatever you are feeling and visualizing in your mind, draw it. This is often a telling and interesting exercise.

Soothing Strategy
Road Map

Draw a map that represents your week. Start with a primary road. Maybe it has hills or turns, straightaways or detours. Label each junction: meeting with the boss to ask for a raise, parent-teacher conference, shopping for groceries, dinner with spouse, niece's birthday party. This map can illuminate your current road to emotional eating. What side streets tempt you most along the way? Is it your anniversary that you're anxious about? Or maybe you know that brunch on Sunday will have your favorite croissants? At the end of the road, draw something to represent emotional eating, like a doughnut. Then go to the beginning and place doughnuts on all the events on the map that you know will be high-temptation events that'll bring on cravings for comfort food. Having a map laid out for your week that clearly identifies problematic events may help you be more aware of them.

Art washes away from the soul the dust of everyday life.
—Pablo Picasso

38. Origami

I was first introduced to the ancient art of origami as a young adult when I was living and studying in Japan. Origami is the Japanese art of folding squares of paper into complex yet beautiful shapes.

After becoming frustrated by my inability to fold things just right and almost giving up, something magical happened: I caught myself experiencing a sense of calm. No longer berating myself for making a mistake, I enjoyed the feeling of serenity that washed over me as I continued to work with the paper. Creating origami provided the intense feeling of being so engrossed in an activity that I lost all track of time, couldn't hold a negative thought in my head, and didn't feel the need to reach for comfort food. For me, origami provided that state of flow where problems, worries, obsessive thoughts, and even the outside world disappeared for a brief time.

In that moment, I finally understood the calming benefits of origami:

- Origami activates both the right and left hemispheres of the brain (Taylor and Tenbrink 2013). As a result, this leads to the development of motor, intellectual, spatial, and creative abilities.

- Origami requires focus, attention, and your full presence. Because your mind is totally engaged in the present moment, this intense concentration distracts you from your cravings—particularly food cravings. This distraction leads to a decrease in feelings of depression, anxiety, and stress.

● Origami enhances your creativity. By tapping in to this outlet for creative expression and relaxation, you'll achieve a sense of accomplishment as you transform that small square of paper into a work of art.

The value of origami is in the process of creating and in the feelings of accomplishment gained by building your skills. Therefore it is important to remain detached from the outcome and not seek others' approval of your work. It is for you! You may also want to keep track of the times when paper folding leads to feelings of calm and relaxation. You might even develop a new, fun hobby. Need help? Watch me demonstrate origami at http://www.eatingmindfully.com/demonstrations.

Soothing Strategy
Make a Paper Crane

When you feel the urge to eat emotionally, or if you are struggling with boredom eating, try making a simple crane. You'll need a square piece of paper. Clear, illustrated directions for the exercise can be found at: http://www.eatingmindfully.com

/demonstrations. After you complete one crane, repeat until the urge to eat passes!

Did you know that many Japanese believe that if you fold 1,000 paper cranes, your wish will come true? These thousand cranes, which are called *senbazuru*, are strung together and hung up. The popularity, in part, comes from a book titled *Sadako and the Thousand Paper Cranes*, by Eleanor Coerr and Ronald Himler. The book brought massive exposure to the origami practice and art. Since the book was published, the paper crane has also become a symbol for peace. If you struggle with emotional eating and wish to get past it, start your own crane chain. In moments of struggle, make another one to add to the chain. It will keep your hands and mind occupied.

Soothing Strategy
Dollar Bill Origami

Don't have a piece of paper? Or are you struggling not to spend your last dollar in the vending machine? From butterflies to bow ties, you can turn your food money into art with a simple one-dollar bill. Get started at: http://www.eatingmindfully.com/demonstrations.

Origami is a metamorphic art form, you got that piece of paper, you don't add to it you don't take away from it, you change it.
—Michael LaFosse

Soothing Your Senses

We experience the world through our senses. On one end of the continuum, we luxuriate in the pleasure of soft sheets, the taste of an exquisite piece of fruit, or the scent of a cinnamon-flavored candle. At the other end, there's sensory pain—touching a hot stove burner, smelling rotten food from an overfilled garbage can, or hearing the jarring noise of a blaring siren.

Consider a time when you were driving in a car and the music was very loud. You likely turned down the dial to a softer, more comfortable volume. In that moment, you felt instant relief. You might have even said, "Ahh." This is an example of a sensory experience that we can control by changing the environment. However, there may be other situations that are out of your control, resulting in negative sensations in which it feels like there's no escape. Picture yourself trapped in a club with blaring disco music when you have a headache, or stuck at a friend's home where incense is burning with an aroma that makes you feel nauseous. You may feel as if the uncomfortable emotions or sensations will last forever—though most of us know that, rationally, this is rarely the case.

Turning to food is one way we soothe our senses. But this is problematic when it leads to overeating. This section of the book provides myriad ways to use your senses in ways other than gorging on food. Skim the Soothing Strategies that follow, then choose the technique that excites you the most. Every few days, introduce a new strategy into your repertoire, and decide which suggestions work best for you. Make it a game—a treasure hunt to find how many ways you can delight and calm your senses, all while minimizing your temptation to engage in emotional eating.

39. Thalassotherapy

Thalassotherapy, from the Greek word for "sea," is a therapy that incorporates the medicinal benefits of seawater. Seawater is purported to have many beneficial effects on the skin and pores, and it produces even more useful benefits as a stress soother. The origins of thalassotherapy may trace back centuries to the Romans, who used warm water and bath "treatments" as medicinal cures. Today we know water-based therapies as *hydrotherapy*, which includes everything from saunas to steam baths, foot baths, and sitz baths; the applications of water compresses; Watsu, a type of meditative massage in water; and flotation therapy, during which you float in a tank of water saltier than that of the Dead Sea to create a restorative neurological state that induces relaxation and serenity and bolsters creativity, among other benefits.

Although you may not live near the sea, that's okay. You can create your own sealike water using Epsom salts. Epsom salts are a mineral compound of magnesium and sulfate. You may remember Epsom salts as a cure your grandpa used once upon a time to soak his calloused feet. The white crystals have seen a comeback in recent years and are touted for everything from reducing inflammation to helping muscles and nerves recover, flushing toxins, and easing headaches, to name a few. One study shows that thalassotherapy is helpful in reducing pain for people who have fibromyalgia (de Andrade et al. 2008).

Jill is a client who struggles with emotional eating. She has fibromyalgia symptoms that cause pain in her joints and muscles. During a flare-up, she would curl on her couch and munch on popcorn and pretzels. It eased her pain for a moment, but in the long run made her feel lethargic, bloated, and guilty about the extra calories consumed. Jill started taking a hot bath with Epsom salts to relax her muscles and create a sense of calm. Not only did the soothing soak alleviate pain, it improved her mood and reduced her urge to snack.

Even if you do not suffer from physical pain, water's power helps us feel relaxed, calm, and energized—and when you operate from a place of serenity you are better able to handle all of life's curveballs, including the temptation to overeat. And best of all, you can overcome emotional eating!

Soothing Strategy
A Soothing Saltwater Soak

Try this hot soak in the tub whenever an urge to eat for comfort hits. Epsom salts will relax muscles and relieve tension.

Run a tub as hot as you can stand it and pour in 2 cups of Epsom salts. If you want a super-soft skin-saver bonus, pour 1/2 cup of olive oil or baby oil in the tub, too. Don't use soap or bubble bath with Epsom salts, as it can interfere with the action of the salts.

If you have a fragrant oil you want to add, pour a few drops in as well.

Sit down in the water and soak at least 15 minutes.

Soothing Strategy
Calming Salt Scrub

If you don't have time for a soak, try adding Epsom salts to your regular shower. The invigorating scrub helps to exfoliate dead skin, detoxify, and provide some of the muscle-relaxing, stress-relieving effects that you receive when you soak in the salts.

After washing in the shower, apply handfuls of Epsom salts to wet skin and scrub lightly. Use the salts over your entire body. Then rinse off.

Towel off and apply a nice, thick moisturizer to retain the smooth-skin effect. It's the next best thing when you don't have time for a longer relaxing soak in the tub.

Soothing Strategy
Sensory Detox

Here is an effective detox based on what happens in a sensory deprivation chamber (a tank filled with warm water for the purpose of soothing overstimulated senses). As an added bonus, this type of bath helps to increase your creativity, as it reduces external noise that your mind has to process. You are left only with your thoughts.

Fill a tub with water. Add 2 cups of Epsom salts. The salts will help you to feel buoyant and weightless. Turn down the lights—or turn them off completely—and reduce the noise level as much as possible (wear earplugs if necessary).

Step into the tub and float for 10 minutes—or however long you need. Set a timer so you don't stress about the clock.

There must be quite a few things that a hot bath won't cure, but I don't know many of them. —Sylvia Plath

40. Aromatherapy

Known as nature's first medicine, essential oils have been used for thousands of years. Their medicinal properties date back some 4,500 years. The Egyptians and Greeks were well acquainted with essential oils and used them for medical, spiritual, and personal purposes. In fact, the Bible mentions essential oils more than 200 times. Remember frankincense and myrrh?

Essential oils are made from the liquid part of shrubs, trees, flowers, roots, stems, fruits, and bark. They are usually produced through a steam distillation process. It may take hundreds of pounds of leaves to produce a highly concentrated, potent oil. Each oil may contain up to 200 different chemical properties, many of which are antimicrobial, antiviral, antifungal, and anti-inflammatory. A very small amount can be used effectively for a variety of emotional, physical, and spiritual symptoms. Different oils can be blended together to create one-of-a-kind tinctures that can be inhaled, applied directly to the skin, or sprayed into the surrounding air or on linens and clothing. Some people even take them internally.

Aromatherapy has proven benefits for dealing with a range of health issues including but not limited to wound care, skin care, digestion, headaches, cancer, high blood pressure, arthritis, asthma, diabetes, and more. Essential oils are particularly useful for dealing with emotions, and because of that they can be excellent tools to help you successfully conquer emotional eating.

Additionally, essential oils can be used to reduce appetite and aid in weight loss due to their ability to stimulate the part of the brain that governs feelings of satiety (fullness after eating).

While essential oils may enter your body through your skin or mouth, they have a direct path to your brain via your nasal passages. As an aroma is inhaled, the molecules are trapped by olfactory membranes in the nose where nerve cells then trigger the olfactory bulb, which processes odors, and send impulses to the limbic system of the brain, which influences hormone balance, blood pressure, breathing, heart rate, emotions, and memory. In other words, while this sounds fairly complicated, it simply means that smelling essential oils stimulates the brain in such a way that they react with bodily systems to kill bacteria and viruses, stimulate the immune system, calm and soothe nerves and anxiety, and augment many other functions.

Does it work? A study of angry drivers found that sniffing the scent of cinnamon and peppermint reduces frustration and increases alertness behind the wheel (Raudenbush et al. 2009). Cinnamon and peppermint resulted in increased alertness and decreased frustration during the course of a frustrating driving scenario. Furthermore, sniffing peppermint scent reduced anxiety and fatigue. The point? Pleasant scents have the power to dramatically impact your mood.

Match the Right Essential Oils to Your Needs

Aromatherapy can help to curb your appetite and calm and soothe anxiety over food issues, quiet the endless food chatter in your mind, improve your digestion, and lighten feelings of hunger and more. I recommend that you arrange for a consultation with a certified aromatherapist, who can concoct a blend of the right oils and find the right delivery method for you. But if an aromatherapist isn't nearby, here's a simple guide for choosing them on your own for whatever your issue is right now:

Uplifting scents: lemon, orange, grapefruit, balsam fir, Idaho blue spruce, nutmeg

Relaxing scents: lavender, valerian, Roman chamomile, ylang-ylang, tangerine, angelica

For indigestion: peppermint, spearmint, fennel, anise, ginger

For hunger: peppermint, spearmint, ocotea, grapefruit

For focus and concentration: jasmine, lemon, basil, peppermint, rosemary

Soothing Strategy
Selecting the Best Therapeutic Oils

While essential oils are readily available over the counter, unfortunately in the United States there are no regulations or certification for the quality of essential oils. Sadly, many essential oil "manufacturers" extend their oils with oils that are not essential oils such as vegetable oils. Synthetic oils made in a laboratory are also sometimes used, as well as chemical extraction processes that produce oils that are less than pure and contain residues that you don't want to put in your body or inhale. Only the highest-grade oils are going to produce reliable therapeutic results. To make sure you get the highest quality oils follow these guidelines:

- Make sure the oil is therapeutic grade.

- Select organic if possible.

- Learn a little about the company you are buying your oils from. Where does it source its oils from? How does it produce the oil? What are its testing procedures? How many years has the company been in the business of producing essential oils?

- A quick test of quality is to see how quickly the oil absorbs into your skin. When essential oil is pure and of high grade, it will absorb into your skin very quickly and will not feel greasy. On the other hand, if the oil has been cut with other oils or substances, it will feel greasy and take a long time to absorb into the skin. So when testing oils, put a drop on your skin and see how much time it takes to absorb.

- Buy quality oils from companies that are GC/MS (gas chromatography/mass spectrometry) tested. This chemical test gives the breakdown of ingredients in a batch of oil. Some less-ethical companies produce "oils" that may be only 20 percent pure oil and 80 percent filler. Companies with pure products can produce a GC/MS report. If a company balks or says it doesn't do that, buy elsewhere.

Soothing Strategy
Seven Ways to Use Essential Oils

Essential oils are nature's gift to your good health. The next time you notice that you're about to eat for emotional reasons, soothe your sense of smell. You'll be pleasantly surprised! Here are some ways to get the most benefit from essential oils:

- Put 1 or 2 drops on your palms, rub your hands together, and cup them over your nose. Take several deep breaths. You can also inhale the oil directly from the bottle. Try orange essential oil to instantly change your mood!

- Use a diffuser, which sends fine particles of the oil into the air that can stay in the environment for hours. This is particularly helpful when faced with challenging emotions or when using oils for weight loss.

- Add 5 to 10 drops of essential oil to your bathwater.

- Put 1 or 2 drops of essential oil on a cotton ball and place it in the vent of your car.

- Use the oils neat—that is to say, put them right on your body. It is always a good idea to test for sensitivity first by putting a drop on the back of your hand and see how you respond. You can also dilute the oil by using a carrier oil, such as almond, jojoba, or olive oil. More powerful oils will require a dilution of 1 part essential oil to 4 parts carrier oil. Other oils may be diluted with equal parts.

- Some essential oils may also be ingested by putting a drop or two in water or into a capsule with a carrier oil. Be sure you are using the highest-quality oils. Try a drop of peppermint oil in a glass of water and see if your urge to eat stops.

- Blend several essential oils with a carrier oil and use it to inhale; or apply it topically, when the urge to soothe yourself with food strikes, when food chatter won't turn off, or when faux hunger pangs hit.

Behave so the aroma of your actions may enhance the general sweetness of the atmosphere. —Henry David Thoreau

41. Creative Visualization

In 1994, actor Jim Carrey wrote himself a fake check for $10 million before he made it big. Just months before the date written on the fake check, he was paid $10 million for a movie role. In interviews, he credits this exercise as a significant part of his success. Being able to "see" what you want has to happen first. Visualization isn't always going to make you a millionaire. But what it can do is help to shape your behaviors to bring you closer to your goals.

Creative visualization works for a variety of reasons. First, it gets you focused on what you really want; it helps you to define your goals, big or small. By reviewing the same message or image day in and day out, you are programming your subconscious mind to respond and act accordingly. All actions begin with thoughts; we have an idea, and then comes the manifestation of that idea. This can happen consciously or unconsciously. By becoming conscious of what you really want and envisioning that goal, you are asking the subconscious and conscious mind to work together, which is very powerful. Further, at a very deep level you could say that everything in our universe is connected. So when you consistently put a certain thought out into the world, the universe responds by giving you what you are asking for. The trick is to be sure you ask for what you really want! Best of all, visualization can help your mind simply relax.

You might think that visualizing food in coping with cravings might be counterintuitive, making the urge worse. Not so, according to a study on M&M's. Researchers asked one group of people to imagine eating three M&M's and putting thirty quarters in a slot. The other group visualized eating thirty M&M's (the amount in one package) and putting thirty quarters in the slot. Then each group was given access to a bowl of actual M&M's and told to help themselves. Interestingly, those who imagined eating thirty M&M's consumed half as many than the group who visualized three M&M's. The researchers hypothesized that the mind acts "as if" something has already happened and responds accordingly (Morewedge, Huh, and Vosgerau 2010).

For instance, if you are imagining a stressful event, your body releases stress hormones as if it's happening right now. Thus, imagining M&M's, if they're something you like, may release dopamine, the chemical that sends a hit of pleasure to the brain. Or it might be due to habituation. It isn't that people enjoy the food less; it's that they spend less effort obtaining it. How can you put this into use? If you are trying to cope with a chocolate craving, closing your eyes and imagining eating chocolate calmly and enjoying it will likely trigger pleasure in your brain. The study was repeated with cheese cubes and the same result was found (Morewedge, Huh, and Vosgerau 2010).

What's more, the study was recently repeated with gummy bears and walnuts (Missbach et al. 2014). It's sort of like an imagination diet. Imagine you ate the delicious cookie, chocolate bar, bowl of ice cream, or your fill-in-the-blank favorite food. Visualize the taste, smell, and texture—enjoying the experience in the fullest. Your mind thinks you already had the experience, and you don't need to eat it anymore. (Interestingly, the approach isn't as effective in those who were depleted or tired, perhaps because you cannot visualize the experience of eating something delicious as effectively as you need to when you are fatigued.)

Here's how visualization worked for one of my clients, Celeste, a thirty-nine-year-old e-mail marketer who works long hours from home. Her desk was like a candy store with drawers overfilled with chocolate and treats. In her first session with me, Celeste stated that her goal was to break loose from emotional eating, although she did not "believe" she could. During the next session, I asked her to do nothing more than close her eyes at night and imagine what it would be like if she broke completely free from emotional eating. I encouraged her to imagine it in great detail: what she would be wearing, what her desk would look like, how she would sit at her desk. In the next session, Celeste said she had an "aha" moment. She had pictured a non–stress eater having a clean desk, wearing a nice outfit, and sitting up straight instead of slouching back in her chair. This image gave her something to work for. The next day, Celeste wore dress pants (instead of her usual sweatpants) and intentionally sat up straight in her chair. She also cleaned off her desk.

Soothing Strategy
Visualizing Mindful Eating

Try these steps to curb emotional eating:

On a piece of paper write out how you would like to eat. Make it your ideal scenario. Maybe it is eating healthier foods, choosing nonfood ways to relax, walking away from too much sugar, or setting the table with cloth napkins and fresh flowers one night a week. Be sure to keep it realistic, obtainable, and positive. If you get stuck, imagine what a nonemotional eater would do and write that down.

During a quiet moment of the day, such as before you go to bed, close your eyes and imagine yourself having achieved the ideal scenario you wrote about. Visualize all of the details, from what you are wearing to the arrangement of food on the plate. Walk yourself through the steps of making choices other than eating during times of stress. How would it feel to successfully negotiate this?

Repeat this exercise many times throughout each day and for at least 30 days to see change.

Soothing Strategy
Display Your Goals

Once you define your goal for creative visualization, another way to use this technique is to create a digital board or other inspiration board. Try using Pinterest or a similar social media site. Assemble a collage of images that represent what it is you're trying to achieve. Pin images, words, or phrases that resonate with you; healthy foods or recipes you want to eat more of; people engaging in fun activities like hiking or playing with children outside; and so on. You can also do it the old-school way with magazine pictures and a corkboard.

Develop your imagination—you can use it to create in your mind what you hope to create in your life.
—Stephen Covey

42. Activate Your Senses

You may find yourself stiff, sore, or drained at the end of the day—and this discomfort can contribute to your desire to eat. Or maybe you can't unwind because your emotions are running high from stress and anxiety, and that's what leads you to the chips and chocolate.

Using the five senses—touch, smell, sight, hearing, and taste—can go a long way to helping you unwind and soothe yourself more naturally. Ever light a candle and feel instant calmness? How about when you slip into a hot, scented bath and feel the tension dissipate? Maybe standing at the precipice of a beautiful nature trail and listening to a bird's song brings relief to your soul. No matter which sense soothes you best, or if it's a combination of all of them, there's a bonanza of soothing to be had when it comes to your senses.

Any uncomfortable feelings in the body may trigger emotional eating. But if you can activate *other* senses—or soothe the bodily sensations that are bothering you in the first place—then you'll find it easier to nurture yourself with these healthier alternatives.

Some of the following exercises will calm and soothe you, while others may help you to feel more energized and upbeat. What all of these techniques have in common is that they will allow you to use your senses to move away from emotional eating as you instead turn toward feelings of well-being and contentment.

Soothing Strategy
Ease and Please the Senses

Here are some common feelings and what you can do about them:

When you're feeling uncomfortable...

- Ease your senses by loosening your clothing and taking off your shoes.

- Please your senses by putting on something soothing to your skin, such as a silk shirt or a soft cashmere sweater.

When you're feeling hot, flushed, or anxious...

- Ease your senses by finding a cooler room, pulling the shades down to darken the room, or turning on a fan.

- Please your senses by drinking some cool lemon- or mint-flavored water to make your taste buds sing.

When you're feeling worried...

- Ease your senses by mentally letting go of your worries. Releasing them is healing. Sit quietly and close your eyes. Inhale and say to yourself, "When I let go of what I am, I might become what I might be" (a quote by Lao Tzu).

- Please your senses by holding an object (a pebble, small ball, or anything else that symbolizes your worry) in your hand and closing your palm around it. With your hand still closed, turn your hand over, and then open it. This is much like emotion: We wrap ourselves around it, holding it tight, attached to it. But you *can* let it go. When the object falls to the floor, you have handed it over for the world to take care of it. You can even use this imagery without actually having an item in your hand. Simply visualize letting go of whatever it is you are feeling, then watch it drop.

When you are feeling angry...

- Ease your senses with balloons. Write down on little pieces of paper your grievances. Stick the paper into several balloons and blow the balloons up. Place all the balloons on the ground.

- Please your senses by stomping on the balloons.

Soothing Strategy
Soothe Your Senses

Here are ideas to push you out of whatever crummy way you're feeling, using all five senses:

- **Sense of sight:** Look all around you and find at least three visual objects that calm you; focus on these objects for a little while. Or dim the lights and notice how different things look. Or mindfully gaze at a calming picture, observe fish swimming in a tank, watch a crackling fireplace, look at crashing ocean waves, or gaze at the clouds. Or if your eyes are tired, soothe them with something cool on your eyelids for 4 to 5 minutes; cool cucumber slices, a cold facecloth, slices of raw potato, a cool tea bag, or even a chilled spoon all work well.

- **Sense of sound:** Turn on some soothing music and relax. Or mindfully listen to the sounds of nature or the sound of children laughing. Or enjoy a moment of silence. What are three other sounds that are music to your ears?

- **Sense of touch:** Find three tactile items that are pleasing to touch; close your eyes and enjoy how they feel. Or put something pleasing on your skin: maybe wrap yourself in a fuzzy blanket or a comfy robe, or wear something made of silk, suede, or velvet. Or try holding a mug of warm coffee or gripping an ice cube.

- **Sense of taste:** Soothe your mouth with a variety of flavors and textures: eat a peppermint, chew cinnamon gum, crunch on an ice cube, drink carbonated water, or simply brush your teeth.

- **Sense of smell:** Identify various scents you enjoy. Perhaps you prefer the scent of essential oils, a cinnamon stick, a dryer sheet, a dab of perfume, a specific flower, or the smell of healthy soup cooking on the stove.

Soothing Strategy
Energy Boosters

Feeling bored? Dragging yourself around? Try one of these energy boosters—without the negative effects or addictive qualities that come from food or lots of caffeine:

- **Stretch your chest.** Stand in the middle of a doorway and place your palms flat against the wall on either side of the doorframe. Make sure your back is straight. Lean forward through the doorway without moving your hands. You should feel a stretch across your chest. Move your hands higher or lower to stretch different areas of your chest.

- **Stretch your arms.** Stand facing a solid wall. Place your right hand flat against the wall, and lift your left leg slightly so that most of your weight is on your standing leg and some weight is supported by the wall through your arm. Tighten your abdominals and keep your back straight. Lightly touch the fingers of your left hand to the armpit of your right arm, then reach out and up until your left arm is reaching straight overhead, fingers pointing toward the ceiling. Keep your right shoulder blade down. Hold for 5 seconds and repeat 10 to 15 times. Switch sides.

- **Breathe faster.** This will get your oxygen pumping.

- **Change your scenery.** Your senses can get accustomed to your surroundings, and simply changing environments can perk them up.

- **Enliven your legs.** Lie on your back and raise one leg and then the other until they are both in the air. Now shake them for a minute or two.

- **Mindfully drink green tea.** A cup of green tea has properties that are proven to boost alertness (Chacko et al. 2010; Yoto et al. 2014).

- **Stand instead of sit.** Sitting is the new smoking—long-term sitting can sabotage your health. Step away from your desk whenever you can, since sitting still for too long can drag you down. Standing up can help counteract the effects of inertia. You can alternate sitting and standing for a minute at a time to get your blood flowing.

- **Chew gum.** Gum has been shown to stimulate the brain waves that ignite concentration and focus. In fact, studies show that chewing gum can shift your brain waves to a state of relaxed alertness (Allen, Jacob, and Smith 2014).

*Every now and then go away, have a little relaxation,
for when you come back to your work your judgment will
be surer. Go some distance away because then the work
appears smaller and more of it can be taken in at a glance,
and a lack of harmony and proportion is more readily seen.*
—Leonardo da Vinci

43. Hypnosis

What do you think of when you hear the word "hypnosis"? You probably visualize a comedy show during which the hypnotist waves a magic pocket watch in front of an audience member's eyes while saying, "You are getting very sleepy." Movies and TV shows have popularized this notion, causing people to have a hard time taking hypnosis seriously, since it's portrayed like a party prank or a trick. But the truth is that self-hypnosis can be a powerful tool for helping you change unwanted thoughts and behaviors. What's more, it's actually initiated by you, and you are in complete control.

There have been several new studies that examine how hypnosis can be used in medical settings, particularly in dealing with anxiety related to medical conditions and procedures. This is called "state-related anxiety." It's when some upcoming event is more situationally related, such as a dentist appointment, labor, or surgery. Hypnosis is also used to help with anxiety-triggered conditions such as tension headaches, irritable bowel syndrome, and those conditions that can spark significant anxiety such as cancer.

The upside of self-hypnosis is that it is free, nonaddictive, chemical-free, and something you can do almost anywhere and anytime. Hypnosis, when done correctly, is thought to change brain waves and help move people into a relaxed state. This is good news for emotional eaters. Often, emotional eaters describe eating as a way to enter a state of emotional void. Think about how mindlessly you munch while watching a television show or reading a book. During hypnosis, you're not asleep. Instead, you are turning on your subconscious mind and putting it to work.

The downside, if there is one, is that self-hypnosis techniques have not been standardized in many studies, and it's difficult to conduct rigorous clinical studies on it. Many published studies end with a request for more to be done to investigate how hypnosis really works or how it helps.

You may actually have entered a state very like hypnosis in the past and not realized it. For example, if you've ever been so totally engrossed in a project that you don't hear someone call your name even when he or she is right next to you, or if you completely lose track of all time when you're engaged in a beloved hobby like quilting or scrapbooking, or if when you're driving you all of a sudden "wake up" and realize that you passed your exit. You were conscious but not fully attuned or using all of your levels of awareness.

Interestingly, many people use food in a self-hypnotic way. Maybe you've been mindlessly munching and all of a sudden realized you ate the whole box of crackers or most of the bowl of popcorn. What we need to change with self-hypnosis is two-fold: learning not to reach for the food mindlessly in the first place; and, when we are enjoying food, staying fully present and aware in the moment.

Soothing Strategy
Counting Down

When in a trancelike state, people are more open to suggestion and less vulnerable to criticism. In this exercise, you'll use this trancelike, open state of mind to bring up suggestions of other, healthier things you can do instead of mindlessly or emotionally eating. Practice at least once every day. One hypnosis session isn't going to conquer all your cravings; repetition and frequent self-hypnosis sessions are essential.

Decide on a blinking pattern for your eyes, and apply while opening and closing your eyes as you count backward. For example, one pattern is to open your eyes on even numbers and close them on odd numbers.

Start at 100 and begin to count backward.

When you land every tenth number (90, 80, 70, and so on) say to yourself, "I eat only when I am hungry" or "When I feel strong emotions, I easily find constructive ways to deal with them" or any mantra that is helpful to you.

When you reach 0, open your eyes and focus back on the room.

Soothing Strategy
Power Place

Self-hypnosis is a powerful tool for helping you change unwanted behaviors like emotional eating. It produces a relaxed state of mind, reduces anxiety, and helps impart a more positive outlook on life. Just remember to practice!

Choose a quiet place.

Close your eyes and tune in to the sounds around you: the hum of a heater, wind, a car driving by outside, a nearby voice, and so on. As you notice these sounds, also notice how your body feels: How do your feet feel against the floor? Or your head against the pillow? Or your thighs against the chair seat? Begin to notice the rhythm of your breath.

As you tune in to your breath, imagine that you are in a kitchen with stairs leading up to an outside terrace. As you mentally take each step, imagine leaving your worries behind. Food and comfort foods are in the refrigerator. With each step, you move farther and farther away from these foods. Mentally turn around and wave good-bye. Then, say an affirming thought such as "I am powerful and in charge of my eating." (Avoid saying a negative thought such as "Cookies will make me fat.") Repeat this affirmation a few times, each time saying it with more and more conviction.

Now begin to notice how you feel in your body, and pay attention to the sounds around you.

Gently open your eyes and come back to the present.

Soothing Strategy
A Recipe for Your Cravings

Open up your mind to healthy ways of coping with your cravings.

Get into a comfortable position. Close your eyes and take a few long, slow breaths.

Think of a time when you usually engage in emotional eating, like after work, on a lonely Sunday afternoon, or after an exasperating call with your mom.

Now, imagine flipping through a recipe card file. On each card, instead of a food recipe, imagine an image with an alternative, nonfood soothing activity, especially one you enjoy. Maybe a nature hike, a swim in the pool, reading a good book, or organizing your messy closet (okay maybe you don't *like* that one, but you get the gist). Truly create a visual of you participating in each activity.

When done, open your eyes and come back to the room. Hopefully, mindlessly eating will be the furthest thing from your attention. Plus, you may actually take yourself up on one of those activities!

Compared to what we ought to be, we are half awake.
—William James

44. Feng Shui

Have you ever entered a store or restaurant and instantly felt calm? Conversely, have you ever entered an establishment—perhaps it was dark and dingy, or too bright and cluttered—and said to yourself, "I've got to get out of here!" My client Roger mentioned this feeling to me. He was antiquing with his wife when they entered a store that was musty and crowded with stuff, which wasn't that unusual, but Roger developed a strange, bad feeling in the store. He didn't like the place, didn't want to be there, and decided he wasn't buying anything there. This kind of thing happens to some people. Your surroundings can profoundly impact your emotions—and, of course, your eating. Fortunately, increasing your awareness of your surroundings can be a terrific way to soothe yourself by using the ancient principles of feng shui (Jeffreys 2000).

So what can feng shui do for you and your comfort eating? It can provide an increased sense of peace and inner harmony. With respect to food, many studies have examined how lighting, noise, and color can impact eating patterns. For example, a recent study found that people enjoyed the experience of drinking wine more if the lighting was red and "sweet" music was playing (Spence and Deroy 2013). Another study found that the color of the plate people eat off of affects how flavorful they perceive their food to be. People in the study were served strawberry mousse on a white or black plate. Those who ate off the white plate found the mousse sweeter, more flavorful, and of higher quality than those who were served on a black plate (Stewart and Goss 2013). It may be the contrast between the color of the food and the color of the plate that matters. A high contrast between the colors (say, a red plate with white rice on it) may make people think the food is better and make them eat more. Whereas a low contrast between food and plate colors makes people eat less. Therefore, you might try a variety of colored plates to see if you notice a difference in appeal or eating behavior.

Feng shui is a wonderful transformational tool that can be used to help change the way a place feels in the same way it made the mousse seem sweeter. Making positive adjustments to your physical environment means that your surroundings are able to support you rather than work against you. To improve your mood without using food, create a special space to go when you need a moment of calm.

The following is a list of ways to bring feng shui into your life. To avoid becoming overwhelmed, try one idea at a time. For example, declutter a small area first. Then experiment with lighting, and later move on to paint, and so forth. Notice which ideas decrease your tendency to comfort eat and which increase feelings of relaxation.

- **Lower the lights—and the volume.** Low lighting and a reduced noise level can decrease stress and increase feelings of well-being. Consider playing a white noise machine, or listen to soothing nature sounds. From CDs to MP3 downloads to streaming (Pandora radio offers numerous nature channels, for instance), the options for infusing some sounds of nature into your daily living space are almost endless.

- **Add blue.** Blue is the most calming color, so repainting your walls can instantly introduce serenity into your living quarters. If you can't (or don't want to) paint the walls, simply add some blue accent colors: blue pillows, a chair with blue upholstery, and so on.

- **Reduce clutter.** Begin decluttering your space by getting rid of old, unwanted, unused items. If you can't stand to throw something out, there are other ways to find a good home for your item: Find a friend who may want it, donate it to an organization like Purple Heart or Goodwill, or sell the item online through Craigslist, eBay, and so on. If you tend to hoard items, start small. Begin with a drawer or room that doesn't have as many items you may be tempted to hold on to. Once you begin to experience the calming effects of clutter-free space, you'll be motivated to tackle the more difficult areas in your home.

- **Create a mindful meditative space.** With a place reserved for meditation, you can find relief from the demands of your hectic life. These simple ideas will get you started: Introduce a fishbowl into your home;

when you need something to focus on, a fish can be the perfect object of your attention. Place a chair next to a window; this will give you a beautiful, clear view of calming clouds. Find a small corner for meditation; this protective space can feel very safe and womblike.

- **Establish active and passive spaces.** Create specific spaces for when you need to be more active such as a workout room or a corner with an easel and paintbrush. And make spaces that are more passive: a cozy chair beneath a reading lamp, a book nook, a comfortable chaise for cuddling.

Soothing Strategy
Feng Shui Yourself Away from the Plate

If you have difficulty putting on the brakes when you start comfort eating, here are some more environmental fixes to curb your eating:

- **Use red plates.** When the mind sees red, it automatically thinks, *stop!* This cue may be just the visual you need to become aware of your comfort eating.

- **Turn up the lights.** Yes, this is a bit contradictory to lowering the lights to feel calmer. But for some, those feelings of tranquility can lead to feeling a bit too relaxed at the dinner table. So if you find yourself in the throes of comfort eating, the brightness is a terrific way to decrease the temptation to linger over your meal (Wansink and van Ittersum 2012), which is a definite possibility when dining by candlelight. One caveat: the brightness may rev up the nervous system, so be careful that you don't begin simply eating more quickly when you turn up the wattage. As an interesting side note, researchers from the University of Arkansas concluded that blue lighting reduces the amount of food men eat (Cho et al. 2015). Even though the lighting didn't alter their willingness to eat, they found that the blue light made the food appear less appetizing.

Manifest plainness, embrace simplicity, reduce selfishness, have few desires. —Lao Tzu

45. Soothing Spices

Spices are, indeed, the "spice of life," as these dried food flavorings possess many health-enhancing properties. Various cultures already understand the importance that spices play in our lives. For instance, the Ayurvedic tradition, a 5,000-year-old system of natural healing in India, reveres spices for its *yogavahi*, or the ability to deliver nutrients to the body's cells. What's more, turmeric is used generously in India thanks to its anti-inflammatory, digestive, and other healing properties. In Thailand, chilies, which contain the compound capsaicin, are used for treating muscle and joint aches as well as boosting metabolism and decreasing caloric intake, and are used as a staple in food to bring heat.

When I was in China, my local guide told me a story about a tomb that had been unearthed and examined in 1972. It had been closed in the second century BCE. One of the major highlights was that the tomb contained many spices that had been used for medicinal reasons. This story and many like it indicate that the use of spices to heal, calm, and soothe is not a new practice. However, it might be a new one to you if you're not currently using spices this way.

Perhaps you use spices to flavor some foods. You sprinkle cinnamon in your oatmeal or on top of your pancakes to boost the flavor. You add oregano and basil to sauces, and flavor chicken with dill or rosemary. While spices help the taste, they also work to help your glucose and lipid levels, reduce inflammation, and lower blood pressure, among many other health advantages, which is why there are endless studies that show us which spice is good for which health complaint. For example, many studies tout cinnamon as a treatment for diabetes (Allen et al. 2013). But even if you don't have diabetes, cinnamon can work wonders for you. It also keeps glucose or blood sugar levels in check and helps improve mood.

In addition to medicinal purposes, seasonings can have an amazing impact on your cravings, mood, and the amount of food you eat; and for these reasons, it's certainly worth your while to consider how spices can benefit you. The following list can help you match several spices with your emotional state so you can avoid the temptation to overeat for physical and/or emotional reasons:

- **For anxiety or nausea:** Try ginger. Your stomach may be upset due to anxiety. Or you may feel bloated, uncomfortable, or nauseous from overeating (Mansour et al. 2012). Sip on a cup of ginger tea, or sprinkle some ginger on your yogurt, milk, or toast. Ginger may suppress appetite when consumed and jump-start sluggish metabolism.

- **For eating healthier:** Try garlic powder. This spice can enhance flavor—and improve health. Garlic is known for boosting your immune system, lowering cholesterol, and thinning your blood (which is great if you are at risk for heart disease). Garlic has been shown to reduce blood pressure, exactly what you need when you're stressed (Wang et al. 2015).

- **For when you're anxious or upset:** Try cinnamon. Cinnamon helps because it lowers blood pressure—something that can skyrocket when you're angry, upset, or anxious. Plus, the mood-elevating properties in cinnamon can boost your spirits naturally. A recent study found that just 2 teaspoons can help lessen the negative effects of eating a fatty meal (Skulas-Ray et al. 2011).

- **For indigestion, gas, or constipation:** Try black pepper. This spice can reduce gas and the symptoms associated with indigestion. Because it increases your body's production of hydrochloric acid, it's less likely that your food will remain undigested and pass into your intestines, leading to unfriendly gut bacteria, which produces gas, irritation, and/or constipation. Black pepper contains a substance called piperine, which has been shown to block the formation of new fat cells (Jwa et al. 2012).

- **For stopping the urge to eat:** Try cayenne pepper. Cayenne can help reduce your appetite by speeding up your metabolism, not to mention kicking up the flavor (which can result in feeling sated more quickly from the pepper's intensity). Another option: Sprinkle some red pepper flakes in a glass of lemon water. The spicy-sour combination is a fantastic way to remain hydrated, with flavor (which has been shown to help reduce appetite too)! Replace your saltshaker with one that has cayenne pepper flakes and find opportunities to sprinkle them on eggs, fish, and more. You can even sprinkle cayenne in your hot chocolate, which is a common practice in Latin America. Adding cayenne pepper to your diet can even reduce your calorie intake by 50 calories a day, since spicy foods fill you up sooner and keep you fuller longer (Janssens, Hursel, and Westerterp-Plantenga 2014).

Spice up your life today! Making spices a daily part of your diet can be tasty and fun, and lessen the temptation to eat for emotional reasons.

Soothing Strategy
Start with Cinnamon

If you don't know where to begin, cinnamon is a great spice to try first because it is probably already in your pantry, has many mood-enhancing qualities, and most people like the taste. If you are feeling edgy today:

- Freeze a few dashes of cinnamon in ice cubes, and then add a few cubes to your water.

- Add a dash either directly into your mug or to coffee grounds before brewing.

- Sprinkle in your tea or onto food such as hot cereal, yogurt, fruit, or granola.

- Mix it into butter for toast, or put it on popcorn.

- Place a few drops in your bathwater. Cinnamon is also known as a warming agent and can help relax and soothe your muscles.

- Add 1 teaspoon of honey and 1/2 teaspoon of cinnamon to boiling water. Sip!

Soothing Strategy
Spice Up Your Life

If there is one day of the week that's routinely difficult—it's your day to run errands, do the kid's carpool, or stay late at night at work, for example—make a dish with a medicinal spice the night before. Then bring leftovers for lunch the next day to buffer the effects of your crazy afternoon. Or if you're planning a night out at a restaurant or creating a meal plan, think ethnic that night; Italian, Mexican, Thai, and Indian foods naturally incorporate spices into their dishes.

I have perfumed my bed with myrrh, aloes, and cinnamon.
—The Bible

46. Mood Tea

Many of us drink liquids in the same way we eat—mindlessly and for comfort—rather than to quench thirst. Plus, many of my clients use coffee and other drinks as an energy replacement to give them a little boost. But research indicates, and my clients tell me, that the right kind of tea can provide both comfort and relaxation without adding empty calories and other substances that aren't good for your mind and body (Bhatti, O'Keefe, and Lavie 2013). The key to finding contentment and using it to deter emotional eating hinges on picking the right tea to match your mood. Different teas provide different benefits. In this chapter, you'll learn which teas can make a huge difference to your mood.

If you live in Europe or Asia, drinking tea is part of your daily life. Tea is the most popular and frequently consumed beverage in the world. But in the United States, tea is not likely to be one of your go-to beverage options. As Japanese scholar and author of *The Book of Tea*, Okakura Kakuzo wrote, "Tea began as a medicine and grew into a beverage."

A review of the benefits of tea reported a laundry list of advantages including reducing inflammation, protecting against a variety of cancers and slowing the growth of tumors, decreasing the risks of heart disease, minimizing the impact of stress, and preventing type 2 diabetes, just to name a few (Bhatti, O'Keefe, and Lavie 2013). In fact, drinking green tea and oolong tea has been associated with a reduced risk of death from a stroke (Mineharu et al. 2011).

How is it that tea can provide all these amazing health benefits? Purists think the best teas—green, black, white, and oolong—contain antioxidant compounds called *flavonoids*, which fight free radicals. And free radicals are molecules that rampage the body, causing oxidative damage, and lead to cancers, heart disease, diabetes, and other health issues. Tea also contains some caffeine and theanine, which are compounds responsible for lifting mood, heightening mental acuity, and providing other mental health benefits.

Some teas help to protect the body from toxins, others aid in alertness, while others help you relax or even sleep. Often, people just pick the type that sounds familiar. But the wrong tea can exacerbate rather than help the problem. For example, too much caffeine can make an anxious person jittery.

Britney, one of my clients, can't sleep because her mind races at night. She thinks about everything she has to get done and obsesses about things that bother her. By morning, she is exhausted and has to drag herself out of bed. She reaches for coffee with a double shot of espresso to try to get through the day. Not surprising, this extreme dose of caffeine leads to higher anxiety and difficulty settling down and focusing at work. So she eats to calm down. Throughout the day she continues to drink coffee too, which leads to an inability to fall asleep again that night. Thus, the cycle continues. Tea would help Britney actually find some calm in the evenings, allowing her mind to settle so she can sleep rather than mask her mood with coffee and reach for food.

Soothing Strategy
Getting the Most out of Tea

Remember: in many cultures drinking tea is a part of everyday life for good reason! Follow the advice of Thich Nhat Hahn, "Drink your tea slowly and reverently, as if it is the axis on which the world earth revolves—slowly, evenly, without rushing toward the future." Here is some more advice:

- **Be mindful.** When do you drink liquids? Is it when you are thirsty, bored, hungry? Start a three-day drinking diary. Create three columns in a notebook or on a blank screen page. At the top of the first column, write "What I drank." At the top of the second column, write "Why I drank it." And in the third, write "How I felt afterward." Be honest. Pay particular attention to column 2, being specific with answers like "because I was thirsty" or "because I was bored" or "because it was offered to me."

- **Consider your mood.** Before you make a cup of tea, assess your mood. Do you need something energizing? Calming? Soothing? Once you determine what you need, consult the next Soothing Strategy section for ideas.

- **Say a mantra.** As you drink, repeat this phrase to yourself: "Refresh, revive, and relax."

- **Build a routine.** Experiment with replacing your morning cup of coffee (if you are a coffee drinker) with tea. Many people find coffee comforting because it is part of their routine. Routine equals comfort. You can keep this routine; just switch your beverage to tea. Consider making 1 cup of tea part of a routine in the morning, afternoon, or evening—whatever is your most vulnerable time for emotional eating. For example, if you often find yourself winding down the evening by eating leftovers or snack foods, try making a nightly tea ritual instead. Ease into your evening with a cup of tea to relax, chill out, and replace the eating habit.

Soothing Strategy
Choosing Tea Based on Your Mood

Tea offers an enormous number of benefits for your body, mind, and emotions. Shopping for tea can be a lot of fun, as is discovering new teas and how they affect you. Experiment and find out which ones bring you balance and peace of mind.

- **For stress:** black tea. Research indicates that black tea can reduce your cortisol (stress hormone) level by 47 percent.

- **For depression and feeling down:** rooibos tea. I recommend this South African herbal tea to my anxious clients due to its soothing properties, in addition to its many health advantages. I also find it calming and helpful in eliminating the desire to emotionally eat. Rooibos tea has been found to help reduce cortisol levels in rats. The researchers hypothesize that this may generalize to humans as well (Schloms et al. 2014), which is great news for emotional eaters. You can find rooibos tea at almost any grocery store.

- **For a queasy stomach, anxiety, or feeling upset:** ginger tea.

- **For sleeplessness and trouble with settling down:** valerian or lavender tea.

- **For feeling too full:** green, oolong, or peppermint tea. You might have heard that green tea is also connected to weight loss. Basically, the properties in green tea help you to burn fat and rev up your metabolism up to 4 percent (Rudelle et al. 2007).

- **For anxiety:** chamomile or lemongrass teas.

- **For boredom or low energy:** chai, black, or green tea. The caffeine helps to kick-start your system and provides alertness. Green tea also contains an amino acid that helps relax your mind without inducing drowsiness.

- **For anger or tension:** white, rooibos, or hibiscus tea. All are reputed to lower blood pressure, which is often raised by stress (Marnewick et al. 2011).

- **For struggles with cravings:** herbal, raspberry, peach, or blueberry tea.

Make tea, not war. —Monty Python

47. Hormonal Balance

I recently interviewed a neuroscientist for one of my *Psychology Today* blog posts to help my followers understand why women crave chocolate during their periods. To date, it has been one of my most popular articles. It's no surprise—women want to know more about this mysterious connection between chocolate and that time of the month. Are the cravings for chocolate and other sweets and comfort foods biological or psychological in nature—maybe both? Approximately 40 to 50 percent of women indicate craving chocolate before their period (Michener et al. 1999). Raise your hand right now if you fall into this category too.

Although the research is unclear regarding the chocolate–PMS connection, there is almost universal agreement concerning the physical and psychological symptoms of PMS itself. You feel awful. Bloated. Tired. Cranky. Food can be momentarily comforting. You have strong cravings for chocolate, salt, or snack foods. Sometimes this leads to a cycle of feeling irritable, overeating, feeling guilty for overeating, experiencing more moodiness, having more cravings—this vicious cycle can frustrate the best of us!

And what about perimenopause? Or menopause? As women enter this phase in their lives, the hormone-related symptoms can be just as debilitating—and sometimes even worse. Interestingly, there is only a slight drop in chocolate cravings post menopause, which suggests that the craving for chocolate and other sweets may not be all hormonally related (Hormes and Rozin 2009).

It may be that when you don't feel good physically, the cognitive restraint (or emotional energy) it takes to say no to your favorite snacks may just be more difficult (Hormes and Timko 2011).

Plus, we may be classically conditioned or evolutionarily programmed to eat sweets and crave good food when we are uncomfortable as a curative, feel-good protective measure. Unfortunately, cavemen didn't have to contend with bags of snack foods or candy bars!

The bottom line is that hormones, and particularly fluctuating hormones, have a powerful impact on your mood and comfort eating. Hormones are an important part of your physiology, from the way you think to what you want to eat to your sex drive. It's no surprise to most women that menopause, perimenopause, pregnancy, and PMS all play a role in comfort eating.

Lower blood levels of zinc, iron, and magnesium have been observed in women with PMS (Chocano-Bedoya et al. 2013). Plus, a recent review of more than sixty herbs, vitamins, and minerals found that only ten were effective in relieving PMS symptoms. You may want to talk to your doctor about adding one or more of these supplements to help you: calcium, chasteberry, vitamin B6, ginkgo, magnesium, pyrrolidone, saffron, Saint-John's-wort, soy, and vitamin E.

Soothing Strategy
Hormone-Balancing Yoga Nidra

A style of yoga that focuses on gentle, supported postures, known as "restorative yoga," has been shown to be highly effective for the symptoms of PMS and menopause as well as for balancing hormones. You will also find that restorative yoga is very relaxing and can be done by almost everyone. One study on yoga nidra, a relaxation-based yoga performed almost entirely in *savasana* (that is, lying down), found that women with abnormal periods who practiced for six months had greater relief from painful symptoms and irregularities than women who didn't take to the mat (Rani et al. 2011). Researchers speculate that the lying down position induced a relaxation response, which allows breathing to slow, the brain to produce more delta waves (similar to sleeping), and the body to drop levels of hormones that may mess up your period.

The following yoga nidra exercise can be practiced for as little as 5 minutes or as long as 30. The longer you take, the more benefit. Enjoy this effortless way to balance your hormones.

Lie down on your back in a comfortable position on a yoga mat, pad, or folded blanket on the floor. Close your eyes and begin to take relaxing breaths.

Bring your attention to your feet, one at a time. Start by relaxing your right foot, noticing any pain or tightness. Then find the most comfortable position to rest it. Next, slowly move your attention to the right knee, thigh, and hip, seeing if there is pain, and consciously relaxing each part on the mat. Repeat with the left leg.

Continue to work up the body: pelvis, stomach, chest, shoulders, each arm, face, and top of head. Intentionally relax each part, breathing into it and focusing on it.

Now take in your entire body as a whole, continuing to enjoy the relaxation.

Slowly turn your head to the right and left. Roll to your right side and rest there a few minutes before slowly sitting up.

Soothing Strategy
Comfort and Care

Here are more ideas for evening out hormones:

- **Turn up the heat.** During your period, your body may feel achy and sore. Use a heating pad to help soothe the aches and pains of cramps. Also, sitting in a warm bath with Epsom salts (see chapter 39, Thalassotherapy) can ease the contractions of the uterus, which are responsible for cramping.

- **Treat the symptoms.** Identify whatever aspect of your period bothers you the most. Too often we shove food at discomfort that can be soothed in other ways. Aim to take care of your particular symptoms. Feel bloated? Avoid salt, too much fiber, and carbonation. Feel uncomfortable in your body or achy? Move mindfully (see the chapters on mindful movement earlier in the book). Omega-3s can be great for helping reduce inflammation and soothing your muscles.

- **Pamper yourself.** Again, look for ways to feel good—soothe your senses with some comfy clothing, spritz essential oils into the air, listen to birds singing.

- **Track your period.** The best way to cope with your period is to not be caught off guard. If you know it's coming, you can get in gear to prepare.

All I really need is love, but a little chocolate now and then doesn't hurt! —Lucy van Pelt

48. Therapeutic Herbs

For thousands of years, civilizations around the world have used herbs for medicinal, nutritional, and cosmetic purposes as well as for spiritual and religious rituals. Today, herbalism is enjoying a popular comeback as more people are looking for natural methods of healing. Learning about herbs is easy with a good book or reputable website, and modern manufacturing and distribution channels make it possible to come by most herbs easily, too.

In simple terms, herbs are plants that offer some type of therapeutic or medicinal property. They might be weeds like daisies, which can be used for digestive problems; spices like cinnamon, which is an uplifting herb; or roots like ginseng, which is particularly good for stress and energy. Additionally, herbs are used for a wide variety of health issues including problems with the immune system, digestion, nervous system, skin, pain, circulation and blood pressure, the reproductive system, and more. They also help with stress management, emotional support, and more.

When available and medically indicated, many of my clients use herbs to get some relief for things like insomnia, anxiety, and stress. They like the idea that they don't add any calories and that they've been used for thousands of years. Herbs are a great supplement to other calming strategies.

Herbs are nature's gift to your good health and calmness. I encourage you to experiment with them—with the permission of your doctor, and some research. They grow wild and you can likely pick or grow your own. Or buy them in capsule or liquid form. There is something beautiful, healing, and calming about growing your own herbs. Or go to your local health food store and explore!

Important note: While most herbs are safe for most people to use, there are certain situations when specific herbs would be contraindicated, particularly if you have an ongoing illness, are on medication, or are elderly. For safety's sake and to achieve the optimum benefit from herbs, I highly recommend that you consult with a qualified herbal practitioner or your health care provider before using any herbs.

Soothing Strategy
Four Ways to Use Lemon Balm

While there are many herbs that help with calming and soothing, lemon balm is particularly helpful and well researched. Lemon balm has been shown to improve mood, relieve stress, and improve cognitive function (Scholey et al. 2014). If you need to relax or calm down, try it! Lemon balm is an easy-to-grow herb and can be found in most stores. *Note:* Lemon balm is not recommended for people with thyroid issues, those who are pregnant, or those taking other medications.

Here are four ideas to get you started:

- **Make lemon balm water.** Fill a jar or pitcher with thinly sliced lemons. Then add lemon balm leaves. Add cold water to the jar, filling it up. It's best and most refreshing if served cold—so place it in the refrigerator for a few hours to brew, then drink a glass cold, straining the leaves.

- **Chew it.** You can chew the leaves directly. Not only will it freshen your breath, it will also release the leaves' calming properties.

- **Infuse your shower.** Get a pair of old panty hose or thin socks. Add lemon balm, rose petals, and lavender, then knot it, making a small sack. Hang it from your tub spout or showerhead, allowing the water to run over it as it fills the tub or while you shower.

- **Get cooking.** Yes, you can also cook with lemon balm. Add it to salads, vinaigrettes, yogurt, and muffins.

Soothing Strategy
Passionflower Tea

Passionflower is another herb that has been clinically tested. It's used as a sleep aid for its soothing and sedative properties. It's reputed to work very quickly to calm you down. Studies show that, in combination with other herbs, passionflower is particularly helpful for relieving tenseness, restlessness, and irritability. It's also been used as an aid to fall asleep (Krenn 2002). If you grow it in your garden, go out and pluck a handful—or buy it from your local health food store or food market.

To make passionflower tea, bring 8 ounces of water to a boil. Put 1 teaspoon of dried passionflower leaves (or 1 tablespoon fresh) in a tea infuser or bag. Place the tea in a cup, add the water, and let steep for approximately 5 minutes. It will make you sleepy, so take it about an hour before bedtime. Limit yourself to 1 cup over a 2-day period.

You can make the tea ahead of time and store in a covered container for when you need it. You can also try mixing 3/4 teaspoon dried passionflower and 1/4 teaspoon dried lemon balm for a different taste.

Note: If you are pregnant, breastfeeding, taking any kind of medication, or operating any machinery, do not drink this.

Lemon balm causeth the mind and heart to become merry.
—Nicholas Culpeper

49. Forest Therapy

Have you ever experienced firsthand the relaxing and rejuvenating calm of a hike along a body of water, a walk in the woods, or a stroll through a peaceful, open green space? In Japan, this activity is called *shinrin-yoku*, or "forest bathing." There, it's a common form of relaxation.

We Westerners may forget about nature's healing powers. That's why I frequently recommend it to clients as an important piece of healing their journey with comfort food. When you have the urge to comfort eat, get out of the kitchen. Fast! Putting food out of arms reach, making it physically less convenient to get to, can be key in interrupting or stopping emotional eating. But forest bathing takes this one step further. Not only are you escaping the kitchen; you're leaving the house, and specifically heading to a calming place in nature that can heal on many levels (Lee et al. 2014).

Intuitively, you may already know this. Who doesn't love to take a walk along the ocean shore, visit a green space in the center of an urban city, or hike through giant redwood trees? Immersing oneself in healing nature is likely responsible for people's desire to hike trails, backpack, ski, swim, walk, run, camp, or participate in virtually any outdoor activity. Research backs it up.

One recent study examined the effect of an urban environment versus a forest environment on physiological dimensions of calm. They found that when people spent time in a forest environment they had a significant decrease in blood pressure, pulse rate, and salivary cortisol concentration (a measure of the stress hormone being produced). In essence, folks were significantly less stressed and more relaxed and calm in the forest environment compared with an urban setting (Song, Ikei, and Miyazaki 2014).

In another study comparing the forest to urban environments, people sat for fifteen minutes while looking out at both settings. Those watching the forest scene felt more calm, relaxed, and rejuvenated—and experienced less anxiety and tension—than those who watched the urban scene for the same fifteen minutes (Ikei et al. 2014). In part, it is the increase in oxygen. You breathe just a little deeper when you are outside. Also, you are disconnected from your computer, away from the bills stacked on your desk and the dishes piled on the kitchen counter.

If you live in an urban area like New York City, San Francisco, or London, you're at higher risk for inactivity and chronic stress, and, as I've noted time and again throughout this book, more stress leads to more emotional eating. This is why people in urban settings should take advantage of their green spaces.

There's even a movement called "environmental neuroscience" that claims people's brains perform better on cognitive tests when they go out in the woods for several days. Just being embedded in nature can improve cognition, physical health, and dozens of emotional complaints. Science is still sorting out exactly how this works, but the theory is that nature pushes your reset button. Apparently, being in a natural setting centers one's equilibrium, reducing stress and all of its effects, from decreasing anxiety and tension to lowering blood pressure, heart rate, and other physical manifestations of stress in the body. Nature centers you. And once you're centered in this way, you may find it easier to rally against food cravings, comfort foods, and emotional eating.

Therefore, it may be of benefit to think about how to reconnect with nature. No matter where you live or work, or what access you have to a natural environment, most everyone can find a small, quiet space in nature to go for a walk or sit and enjoy the surroundings. Try the following strategies when a craving hits or comfort foods are calling.

Soothing Strategy
Forest Bathing

To prevent emotional eating, induce a relaxation response by taking a short hike into a natural setting: a forested area, canyon, beach, garden, or even a nature path in a park. Of course, stay safe, don't go alone, and take precautions in isolated areas. In the study mentioned above, participants walked only 12 to 15 minutes to obtain a sense of calm. You don't have to spend the entire day out there to benefit.

Soothing Strategy
Meditate on Nature

Many people become mindful and move into a meditative moment when they are in nature, whether they realize it or not. Think of a time when you've been at the beach and you stopped to take in the sound of the waves or paused to look at the sun dipping down over the sky. You were likely meditating, however fleeting the moment.

Tune in to the air on your face. Feel the heat of the sun on your skin. It's likely that your mind may want to wander away. Remind yourself that that's okay. Gently nudge your attention back to the environment around you.

If you don't have time to immerse yourself in the outdoors or even go for a walk outside, simply take a look at nature instead. Notice the types of leaves outside your window. Look for birds. Notice any squirrels or wildlife. Or pay attention to the wind and the blue sky above the buildings.

Soothing Strategy
Bring the Forest Indoors

Capture the scents of the forest by lighting a woodsy-smelling candle. Or start a fire in the fireplace, burn incense, or put flowers or other greenery in a vase to enjoy.

I go to nature to be soothed and healed, and to have my senses put in order. —John Burroughs

50. Sex

Why is sex soothing? In part, the act itself is biologically hard-wired in us. Think about it: we probably wouldn't consider having sex if there wasn't some evolutionary emotional benefit to it or if it didn't feel good. That's because when you have sex, sex and orgasms result in increased levels of the hormone *oxytocin*, essentially the "love" hormone, which helps you feel connected to your partner, more bonded, and experience more empathy (Brody 2010).

That's why make-up sex is so common. Not only does it feel good, but the act itself reaffirms the couple's connection, bonds them deeply to one another, and helps restore ill will or negative energy left over from the tiff. Not to mention the release of those hormones makes both of you feel warm and fuzzy toward one another again.

But it doesn't end there. The benefits of sexual activity also include (Brody 2010):

- **Decreased blood pressure:** This is true especially following intercourse or other intimacy.

- **Better sleep:** The endorphins released during sex also help you to feel better, relax, and ultimately get to sleep without worry, stress, and anxiety.

- **Benefits of exercise:** Between the feel-good chemicals you receive in the brain from having sex and the calories burned, think of sex basically as exercise without the treadmill or the expensive gym membership!

Another benefit of sex is that it helps to bring us into the moment, to become present with what is happening right now. This is essential to overcoming negative mind states and the urge to comfort eat.

Of course, people vary in their readiness to become intimate with another person, especially if there are food issues or feelings of self-consciousness involved. And it's not the be-all end-all to weight loss, of course—you can't solve all your food cravings by going out and enjoying sex. In certain situations and for some people, sex can create a lot of anxiety. It can also feel so good that it becomes unhealthy, almost addictive. If this describes you, that's okay. You can utilize other techniques that will work just as well. However, before you completely skip this section, it's important to note that intimacy doesn't always have to lead to orgasm to feel good; this technique still works even with less sexually charged activities. For example, kissing, hand-holding, hugging, and other close physical contact with someone can work just as well. Even reading a romantic novel can stimulate a sexual response!

Always keep in mind that it's important not to have sex when you don't want to. So if you are not in a safe relationship or are too stressed out, this might not be the right technique for you at this moment. But if you are in a satisfying relationship, enjoy it. After all, if you could soothe yourself with warm, intimate contact with someone you care about, or eat some soggy leftover pizza from the fridge, which sounds better?

Soothing Strategy
Soothing Massage

If you are in a loving, committed relationship and feel that sex could be comforting and soothing to you, give it a try. Start by relaxing with 5 minutes of massage for both partners.

One simple technique for couples is to begin with the head, and then work your way down the body. Simply massage your partner's scalp (similar to the motion you use while shampooing), and then use the same gentle, circular motion on your partner's forehead, neck, shoulders, back, buttocks, legs, and feet. You may wish to use massage oil, too. By keeping the lights dim, you'll create the perfect ambience for a relaxing couples' massage!

Soothing Strategy
Getting In the Mood

If you're not in a relationship, or if you feel too self-conscious about your body to imagine sex as a soother right now, you can try reading romantic or erotic stories, or even viewing romantic movies. For instance, Harlequin publishes many series of books that tap in to the romantic side of intimacy. The erotic novel *50 Shades of Grey* and its sequels didn't sell more than a hundred million copies for nothing. If a feel-good romantic movie or a classic romantic comedy gives you a warmhearted, tingly feeling, go for it.

Soothing Strategy
Kiss Someone!

Research suggests that kissing releases chemicals that ease hormones associated with stress, like cortisol (De Boer, van Buel, and Ter Horst 2012). Believe it or not, kissing also gets all your feel-good hormones—serotonin, dopamine, and oxytocin—flowing. These are the same chemicals you can get from exercising, resulting in that little high you get from working out.

Love is an ice cream sundae, with all the marvelous coverings. Sex is the cherry on top. —Jimmy Dean

Best Wishes

Here we are at the end of the book! I'm grateful for the time we've spent together. Thank you for allowing me to share these strategies with you. Taking charge of emotional and comfort eating is something I did, something my clients do every day, and something *you* can do, too. I wish you all the best in your journey going forward!

I also want to thank you for taking this journey with me and allowing me to share both my personal knowledge and professional experience of helping hundreds of clients throughout the years. I'm grateful to be able to share what I've learned to help each of you take charge of your food habits, make healthier food choices, learn to self-soothe in more suitable ways, and discover interesting, fresh, and inspiring methods that hopefully will add dimension, pleasure, and productivity to your busy life.

I hope that you have been patient and gentle with yourself as you moved through the book, discovering new methods of calming and comforting yourself. Some of you may have been using food to soothe for many years, and making the change is like breaking a habit. It's absolutely doable but may not always feel easy without some gentle reminders. This is not the time to beat yourself up because you're not perfect but to treat yourself with positive reinforcement, kindness, and compassion. Please pass this message along to a friend, family member, or other loved one so that they can be part of your mission to change your relationship to food.

If you would like to learn more about my mindful eating programs and the other resources I have created, please check out the original *50 Ways to Soothe Yourself Without Food*, and visit my website http://www.eatingmindfully.com. I hope to see you there!

Mindfully yours,

Susan Albers, PsyD
Cleveland, Ohio

Acknowledgments

A lot of amazing changes took place this year—and I have several humble and heartfelt thank-yous to extend to those who took the major leap forward with me! For fourteen years, I've been writing simply for the sheer pleasure of teaching other people about mindful eating. This year, my message got out wider and bigger than I ever imagined it would—reaching hundreds of thousands of people across the world!

It was my pleasure to create and host the first annual Mindful Eating Summit. I interviewed more than twenty of my favorite eating experts, including many researchers I've admired, colleagues I've e-mailed over the years but have never met, and clinicians who help people to eat more mindfully on a daily basis. A sincere thank-you to these very wise and amazing professionals: Dr. Brian Wansink, Dr. David Katz, Evelyn Tribole,

Dr. Jim Painter, Margaret Floyd, Dr. Elisha Goldstein, Dr. Lilian Cheung, Elisa Zied, Megrette Fletcher, Marsha Hudnall, Dr. Daniel Siegel, Dr. Rick Hanson, Vicki Shanta Retelny, Jennifer Sygo, Cynthia Sass, Dr. Ronald Siegel, Dr. Jean Kristeller, Dr. Nina Savelle-Rocklin, Mary Dye, Dr. Michael Dow, Joe Tatta, Elaine DeSantos, Jonathan Bailor, Dr. Alan Christianson, Dr. Gretchen Rubin, Dr. Nicole Beurkens, Dr. Susan Heitler, Gina Homolka, Dr. Hyman, Dr. Oz, Dr. Barbara Rolls, Marion Nestle, Susan Heady, Dr. Victoria Gould, and many more! Thank you to Trudy Scott, host of the Anxiety Summit, for sharing her insights on how to run an amazing event.

Thank you to Celeste Fine, an amazing literary agent and incredibly smart lady, and her colleagues at Sterling Lord Literistic! Many thanks for the introduction to J. J. Virgin and Dr. Sara Gottfried, who have been incredible role models in getting my message out into the world. Thank you to Camper Bull for introducing me to Bjorn Allpas. I can't thank Bjorn enough for his technical and marketing support. I'd also like to thank Howard VanEs, Jamie Heidel, Jennifer Nelson, and Justin Premick for their valuable contributions to various mindful eating projects.

A special thanks to fellow College of Wooster alumna Chelsea Denlinger for her amazing social media assistance. She is extremely knowledgeable about mindful eating and dedicated to spreading the word! Thank you to Martha Stutzman of All Occasion Photography for her amazing photographs.

Thank you to the team at New Harbinger Publications, particularly Catharine Meyers, Amy Shoup, Tesilya Hanauer, Katie Parr, Jesse Burson, Bridget Kinsella, Heather Garnos, and my editor, Marisa Solís. I started writing with New Harbinger more than fourteen years ago, and here we are. Cheers to many more books on mindfulness!

It has been a pleasure to work at the Cleveland Clinic Family Health Center for over eleven years. What an amazing group of professionals in Wooster! I am appreciative of my fantastic clients, who teach me a lot about emotional eating and generously share their best tips. Readers and fans are also top on my list to thank for their wonderful feedback.

Many thanks to the Wooster crew who joined us in November to celebrate twenty years of friendship. Thank you to my travel buddies: Eric Lingenfelter and Dr. Bronwyn Wilke, Dr. Eric Barr and Heather Barr, and John Bowling. I can't wait for our next adventure. I look forward every year to a fun weekend full of food tours, wine, and chatting with my longtime friends Jane Lindquist Lesniewski and Betsy Beyer Swope. Thank you to Tricia James for running with me late in the evening and listening to my book talk. As always, a special thank-you to Angela Albers and Linda Serotta, Thomas and Carmela Albers, and Rhonda, John, and Jimmer Bowling.

Love and kisses to my favorite calm and comforting crew: John, Jack, and Brooklyn.

References

Allen, A. P., T. J. Jacob, and A. P. Smith. 2014. "Effects and After-Effects of Chewing Gum on Vigilance, Heart Rate, EEG, and Mood." *Physiological Behavior 133,* 244: 251.

Allen, R. W., E. Schwartzman, W. L. Baker et al. 2013. "Cinnamon Use in Type 2 Diabetes: An Updated Systematic Review and Meta-Analysis." *Annals of Family Medicine 11*(5): 452–459.

Bains, G. S., L. S. Berk, N. Daher et al. 2014. "The Effect of Humor on Short-Term Memory in Older Adults: A New Component for Whole-Person Wellness." *Advanced Mind Body Medicine 28*(2): 16–24.

Bhatti, S. K., J. H. O'Keefe, and C. J. Lavie. 2013. "Coffee and Tea: Perks for Health and Longevity?" *Current Opinion in Clinical Nutrition and Metabolic Care 16*(6): 688–697.

Bohns, V. K., and S. S. Wiltermuth. 2011. "It Hurts When I Do This (Or You Do That): Posture and Pain Tolerance." *Journal of Experimental Social Psychology 48*(1): 341–345.

Bongers, P., A. Jansen, R. Havermans et al. 2013. "Happy Eating: The Underestimated Role of Overeating in a Positive Mood." *Appetite 67*: 74–80.

Bonura, K. B., and G. Tenenbaum. 2014. "Effects of Yoga on Psychological Health in Older Adults." *Journal of Physical Activity and Health 11*(7): 1334–1341.

Braude, L., and R. J. Stevenson. 2014. "Watching Television While Eating Increases Energy Intake: Examining the Mechanisms in Female Participants." *Appetite 76*: 9–16.

Brody, S. 2010. "The Relative Health Benefits of Different Sexual Activities." *Journal of Sexual Medicine 7*(4 Pt 1): 1336–1361.

Bushman, B. J., M. C. Wang, and C. A. Anderson. 2005. "Is the Curve Relating Temperature to Aggression Linear or Curvilinear? Assaults and Temperature in Minneapolis Reexamined." *Journal of Personal and Social Psychology 89*(1): 62–66.

Carney, D. R., A. J. Cuddy, and A. J. Yap. 2010. "Power Posing: Brief Nonverbal Displays Affect Neuroendocrine Levels and Risk Tolerance." *Psychological Science 21*(10): 1363–1368.

Chacko, S. M., P. T. Thambi, R. Kuttan et al. 2010. "Beneficial Effects of Green Tea: A Literature Review." *Chinese Medicine 5*: 13.

Chapman, C. D., V. C. Nilsson, and H. Å. Thune et al. 2014. "Watching TV and Food Intake: The Role of Content." *PLoS One 9*(7): e100602.

Chiesa, A. 2010. "Vipassana Meditation: Systematic Review of Current Evidence." *Journal of Alternative and Complementary Medicine, 16*(1): 37–46.

Cho, S., A. Han, M. H. Taylor et al. 2015. "Blue Lighting Decreases the Amount of Food Consumed in Men, but Not in Women." *Appetite 85*: 111–117.

Chocano-Bedoya, P. O., J. E. Manson, S. E., Hankinson et al. 2013. "Intake of Selected Minerals and Risk of Premenstrual Syndrome." *American Journal of Epidemiology 177*(10): 1118–1127.

Church, D., and A. J. Brooks. 2010. "The Effect of a Brief EFT (Emotional Freedom Techniques) Self-Intervention on Anxiety, Depression, Pain and Cravings in Healthcare Workers." *Integrative Medicine: A Clinician's Journal 6*: 40–44.

Cutton, D. M., and C. M. Hearon. 2014. "Self-Talk Functions: Portrayal of an Elite Power Lifter." *Perceptual and Motor Skills 119*(2): 478–494.

Dalen, J., B. W. Smith, B. M. Shelley et al. 2010. "Pilot Study: Mindful Eating and Living (MEAL), Weight, Eating Behavior, and Psychological Outcomes Associated with a Mindfulness-Based Intervention for People with Obesity." *Complementary Therapies in Medicine 18*(6): 260–264.

Danilenko, K. V., S. V. Mustafina, and E. A. Pechenkina. 2013. "Bright Lights for Weight Loss: Results of a Controlled Crossover Trial." *Obesity Facts 6*(1): 28–38.

Danilenko, K. V., I. L. Plisov, M. Hébert et al. 2008. "Influence of Timed Nutrient Diet on Depression and Light Sensitivity in Seasonal Affective Disorder." *Chronobiology International 25*(1): 51–64.

de Andrade, S. C., R. F. de Carvalho, A. S. Soares et al. 2008. "Thalassotherapy for Fibromyalgia: A Randomized Controlled Trial Comparing Aquatic Exercises in Sea Water and Water Pool." *Rheumatology International 9*(2): 147–152.

de Boer, A., E. M. van Buel, and G. J. Ter Horst. 2012. "Love Is More Than Just a Kiss: A Neurobiological Perspective on Love and Affection." *Neuroscience 201*: 114–124.

Dechamps, A., B. Gatta, I. Bourdel-Marchasson et al. 2009. "Pilot Study of 10-Week Multidisciplinary Tai Chi Intervention in Sedentary Obese Women." *Clinical Journal of Sport Medicine 19*(1): 49–53.

Edwards, J. S., H. L. Hartwell, and L. Brown. 2010. "Changes in Food Neophobia and Dietary Habits of International Students." *Journal of Human Nutrition and Diet 23*(3): 301–311.

Fiegel, A., J. F. Meullenet, R. J. Harrington et al. 2014. "Background Music Genre Can Modulate Flavor Pleasantness and Overall Impression of Food Stimuli." *Appetite 76*: 144–152.

Field, T. 2014. "Massage Therapy Research Review." *Complementary Therapies in Clinical Practice 20*(4): 224–229.

Finzi, E., and N. E. Rosenthal. 2014. "Treatment of Depression with Onabotulinumtoxina: A Randomized, Double-Blind, Placebo Controlled Trial." *Journal of Psychiatric Research 52*: 1–6.

Fogarty, S., L. Stojanovska, D. Harris et al. 2015. "A Randomised Cross-Over Pilot Study Investigating the Use of Acupuncture to Promote Weight Loss and Mental Health in Overweight and Obese Individuals Participating in a Weight-Loss Program." *Eating and Weight Disorders*. Advance online publication. doi:10.1007/s40519-014-0175-7.

Germer, C. K., and K. D. Neff. 2013. "Self-Compassion in Clinical Practice." *Journal of Clinical Psychology 69*(8): 856–867.

Godfrey, K. M., L. C. Gallo, and N. Afari. 2015. "Mindfulness-Based Interventions for Binge Eating: A Systematic Review and Meta-analysis." *Journal of Behavioral Medicine 38*(2): 348–362.

Granath, J., S. Ingvarsson, U. von Thiele et al. 2006. "Stress Management: A Randomized Study of Cognitive Behavioural Therapy and Yoga." *Cognitive Behavioral Therapy 35*(1): 3–10.

Gray, C. M., A. W. Tan, N. P. Pronk et al. 2002. "Complementary and Alternative Medicine Use Among Health Plan Members: A Cross-Sectional Survey." *Effective Clinical Practice 5*(1): 17–22.

Holmes, E. A., C. R. Brewin, and R. G. Hennessy. 2004. "Trauma Films, Information Processing, and Intrusive Memory Development."

Journal of Experimental Psychology: General 133(1): 3–22. Retrieved from http://www.apa.org/pubs/journals/releases/xge-13313.pdf.

Hormes, J. M., and P. Rozin. 2009. "Perimenstrual Chocolate Craving: What Happens After Menopause?" *Appetite 53*(2): 256–259.

Hormes, J. M., and C. A. Timko. 2011. "All Cravings Are Not Created Equal: Correlates of Menstrual Versus Non-Cyclic Chocolate Craving." *Appetite 57*(1): 1–5.

Ikei, H., C. Song, T. Kagawa et al. 2014. "Physiological and Psychological Effects of Viewing Forest Landscapes in a Seated Position in One-Day Forest Therapy Experimental Model." *Nihon Eiseigaku Zasshi 69*(2): 104–110.

Janssens, P. L., R. Hursel, and M. S. Westerterp-Plantenga. 2014. "Capsaicin Increases Sensation of Fullness in Energy Balance, and Decreases Desire to Eat After Dinner in Negative Energy Balance." *Appetite 77*: 44–49.

Javnbakht, M., R. Hejazi Kenari, and M. Ghasemi. 2009. "Effects of Yoga on Depression and Anxiety of Women." *Complementary Therapies in Clinical Practice 15(2)*: 102–104.

Jeffreys, P. 2000. "Feng Shui for the Health Sector: Harmonious Buildings, Healthier People." *Complementary Therapy and Nursing Midwifery 6*(2): 61–65.

Jeong Y. J., S. C. Hong, M. S. Lee et al. 2005. "Dance Movement Therapy Improves Emotional Responses and Modulates Neurohormones in Adolescents with Mild Depression." *The International Journal of Neuroscience 115*(12): 1711–1720.

Joshi, M., and S. Telles. 2008. "Immediate Effects of Right and Left Nostril Breathing on Verbal and Spatial Scores." *Indian Journal of Physiological Pharmacology 52*(2): 197–200.

Joshi, M., and S. Telles. 2009. "A Nonrandomized Non-Naive Comparative Study of the Effects of Kapalabhati and Breath Awareness on Event-Related Potentials in Trained Yoga Practitioners." *Journal of Alternative and Complementary Medicine 15*(3): 281–285.

Jwa, H., Y. Choi, U. H. Park et al. 2012. "Piperine, an LXRα Antagonist, Protects Against Hepatic Steatosis and Improves Insulin Signaling in Mice Fed a High-Fat Diet." *Biochemical Pharmacology 84*(11): 1501–1510.

Kalyani, B. G., G. Venkatasubramanian, R. Arasappa et al. 2011. "Neurohemodynamic Correlates of 'OM' Chanting: A Pilot Functional Magnetic Resonance Imaging Study." *International Journal of Yoga 4*(1): 3–6.

Khalsa, D. S., D. Amen, C. Hanks et al. 2009. "Cerebral Blood Flow Changes During Chanting Meditation." *Nuclear Medicine Communications 30*(12): 956–961.

Killingsworth, M. A., and D. T. Gilbert. 2010. "A Wandering Mind Is an Unhappy Mind." *Science 330*: 932.

Kinser, P. A., C. Bourguignon, D. Whaley et al. 2013. "Feasibility, Acceptability, and Effects of Gentle Hatha Yoga for Women with Major Depression: Findings from a Randomized Controlled Mixed-Methods Study." *Archives of Psychiatric Nursing 27*(3): 137–147.

Kraft, T. L., and S. D. Pressman. 2012. "Grin and Bear It: The Influence of Manipulated Facial Expression on the Stress Response." *Psychological Science 23*(11): 1372–1378.

Krenn, L. 2002. "Passionflower (*Passiflora incarnata l.*): A Reliable Herbal Sedative." *Wiener medizinische Wochenschrift 152*(15–16): 404–406.

Kross, E., E. Bruehlman-Senecal, J. Park et al. 2014. "Self-talk as a Regulatory Mechanism: How You Do It Matters." *106*(2): 304–324. doi:10.1037/a0035173.

Kuijer, R. G., and J. A. Boyce. 2014. "Chocolate Cake: Guilt or Celebration? Associations with Healthy Eating Attitudes, Perceived Behavioural Control, Intentions and Weight-Loss." *Appetite 74*: 48–54.

Laing, B. Y., C. M. Mangione, C-H. Tseng et al. 2014. "Effectiveness of a Smartphone Application for Weight Loss Compared with Usual Care in Overweight Primary Care Patients: A Randomized, Controlled-Trial Smartphone Application for Weight Loss in Overweight Primary Care Patients." *Annals of Internal Medicine 161*(10): S5–S12.

Lee, J., Y. Tsunetsugu, N. Takayama et al. 2014. "Influence of Forest Therapy on Cardiovascular Relaxation in Young Adults." *Evidence-Based Complementary and Alternative Medicine 69*(2): 104–110.

Lepp, A., J. E. Barkley, and A. C. Karpinski. 2014. "The Relationship Between Cell Phone Use, Academic Performance, Anxiety, and Satisfaction with Life in College Students." *Computers in Human Behavior 31*: 343–350.

Li, G., H. Yuan, and W. Zhang. 2014. "Effects of Tai Chi on Health Related Quality of Life in Patients with Chronic Conditions: A Systematic Review of Randomized Controlled Trials." *Complement Therapies in Medicine 22*(4): 743–755.

Logel, C., and G. L. Cohen. 2012. "The Role of the Self in Physical Health: Testing the Effects of a Values-Affirmation Intervention on Weight Loss." *Psychological Science 23*(1): 53–55.

Macht, M., and J. Mueller. 2007. "Immediate Effects of Chocolate on Experimentally Induced Mood States." *Appetite 49*(3): 667–674.

Macht, M., S. Roth, and H. Ellgring. 2002. "Chocolate Eating in Healthy Men During Experimentally Induced Sadness and Joy." *Appetite 39*(2): 147–158.

Mansour, M. S., Y. M. Ni, A. L. Roberts et al. 2012. "Ginger Consumption Enhances the Thermic Effect of Food and Promotes Feelings of Satiety Without Affecting Metabolic and Hormonal Parameters in Overweight Men: A Pilot Study." *Metabolism 61*(10): 1347–1352.

Mantzios, M., and J. C. Wilson. 2014. "Making Concrete Construals Mindful: A Novel Approach for Developing Mindfulness and Self-Compassion to Assist Weight Loss." *Psychological Health 29*(4): 422–441.

Marnewick, J. L., F. Rautenbach, I. Venter et al. 2011. "Effects of Rooibos (*Aspalathus linearis*) on Oxidative Stress and Biochemical Parameters in Adults at Risk for Cardiovascular Disease." *Journal of Ethnopharmacology 133*(1): 46–52.

McDaniel, B. T., and S. M. Coyne. 2014. "Technoference: The Interference of Technology in Couple Relationships and Implications for Women's Personal and Relational Well-Being." *Psychology of Popular Media Culture.* Retrieved from http://dx.doi.org/10.1037/ppm0000065.

McVay, M., A. L. Copeland, H. S. Newman et al. 2012. "Food Cravings and Food Cue Responding across the Menstrual Cycle in a Non-Eating Disordered Sample." *Appetite 59*(2): 591–600.

Michener, W., P. Rozin, E. Freeman et al. 1999. "The Role of Low Progesterone and Tension as Triggers of Perimenstrual Chocolate and Sweets Craving: Some Negative Experimental Evidence." *Physiology and Behavior 67*(3): 417–420.

Mineharu, Y., A. Koizumi, Y. Wada et al. 2011. "Coffee, Green Tea, Black Tea and Oolong Tea Consumption and Risk of Mortality from Cardiovascular Disease in Japanese Men and Women." *Epidemiological Community Health 65*(3): 230–240.

Missbach, B., A. Florack, L. Weissmann et al. 2014. "Mental Imagery Interventions Reduce Subsequent Food Intake Only When Self-Regulatory Resources Are Available." *Frontiers in Psychology 28*(5): 1391.

Morewedge, C. K., Y. E. Huh, and J. Vosgerau et al. 2010. "Thought for Food: Imagined Consumption Reduces Actual Consumption." *Science 330*(6010): 1530–1533.

Mrazek, M. D., M. S. Franklin, D. T. Phillips et al. 2013. "Mindfulness Training Improves Working Memory Capacity and GRE

Performance While Reducing Mind Wandering." *Psychological Science* *24*(5): 776–781.

Naghshineh, S., J. P. Hafler, A. R. Miller et al. 2008. "Formal Art Observation Training Improves Medical Students' Visual Diagnostic Skills." *Journal of General Internal Medicine 23*(7): 991–997.

Neal, D. T., W. Wood, and A. Drolet. 2013. "How Do People Adhere to Goals When Willpower Is Low? The Profits (and Pitfalls) of Strong Habits." *Journal of Personality and Social Psychology 104*(6): 959–975.

Nevanperä, N. J., L. Hopsu, E. Kuosma et al. 2012. "Occupational Burnout, Eating Behavior, and Weight Among Working Women." *American Journal of Clinical Nutrition 95*(4): 934–943.

Newberg, A. B., N. Wintering, D. S. Khalsa et al. 2010. "Meditation Effects on Cognitive Function and Cerebral Blood Flow in Subjects with Memory Loss: A Preliminary Study." *Journal of Alzheimer's Disease 20*(2): 517–526.

Obesity Society. 2014. "Thinking about the Long-Term Impact of Your Food Choices May Help Control Food Cravings." *Science Daily* Nov. 4. Retrieved from http://www.sciencedaily.com/releases/2014/11/141104121118.htm.

Oh, H., and A. G. Taylor. 2012. "Brisk Walking Reduces Ad Libitum Snacking in Regular Chocolate Eaters During a Workplace Simulation." *Appetite 58*(1): 387–392.

Oh, H., and A. G. Taylor. 2013. "A Brisk Walk, Compared with Being Sedentary, Reduces Attentional Bias and Chocolate Cravings among Regular Chocolate Eaters with Different Body Mass." *Appetite 71*: 144–149.

Pal, G. K., A. Agarwal, S. Karthik et al. 2014. "Slow Yogic Breathing Through Right and Left Nostril Influences Sympathovagal Balance, Heart Rate Variability, and Cardiovascular Risks in Young Adults." *North American Journal of Medical Sciences 6*(3): 145–151.

Pinaquy, S., H. Chabrol, C. Simon et al. 2003. "Emotional Eating, Alexithymia, and Binge-Eating Disorder in Obese Women." *Obesity Research 11*(2): 195–201.

Polivy, J., and C. P. Herman. 1999. "Distress and Eating: Why Do Dieters Overeat?" *International Journal of Eating Disorders 26*(2): 153–164.

Raghuraj, P., and S. Telles. 2008. "Immediate Effect of Specific Nostril Manipulating Yoga Breathing Practices on Autonomic and Respiratory Variables." *Applied Psychophysiology and Biofeedback 33*(2): 65–75.

Rani, K., S. C. Tiwari, U. Singh et al. 2011. "Six-Month Trial of Yoga Nidra in Menstrual Disorder Patients: Effects on Somatoform Symptoms." *Industrial Psychiatry Journal 20*(2): 97–102.

Raudenbush, B., R. Grayhem, T. Sears et al. 2009. "Effects of Peppermint and Cinnamon Odor Administration on Simulated Driving Alertness, Mood, and Workload." *North American Journal of Psychology 11*(2): 245–256.

Roberts, C. J., I. C. Campbell, and N. Troop. 2014. "Increases in Weight During Chronic Stress Are Partially Associated with a Switch in

Food Choice Towards Increased Carbohydrate and Saturated Fat Intake." *European Eating Disorders Review 22*(1): 77–82.

Roberts, C., N. Troop, F. Connan, et al. 2007. "The Effects of Stress on Body Weight: Biological and Psychological Predictors of Change in BMI." *Obesity 15*(12): 3045–3055.

Rock, M., L. McIntyre, and K. Rondeau. 2009. "Discomforting Comfort Foods: Stirring the Pot on Kraft Dinner and Social Inequality in Canada." *Agriculture and Human Values 26*(3): 167–176.

Rudelle, S., M. G. Ferruzzi, I. Cristiani et al. 2007. "Effect of a Thermogenic Beverage on 24-Hour Energy Metabolism in Humans." *Obesity 15*(2): 349–355.

Skulas-Ray, A. C., P. M. Kris-Etherton, D. L. Teeter et al. 2011. "A High Antioxidant Spice Blend Attenuates Postprandial Insulin and Triglyceride Responses and Increases Some Plasma Measures of Antioxidant Activity in Healthy, Overweight Men." *The Journal of Nutrition* 141(8): 1451–1457.

Schloms, L., C. Smith, K. H. Storbeck et al. 2014. "Rooibos Influences Glucocorticoid Levels and Steroid Ratios in Vivo and in Vitro: A Natural Approach in the Management of Stress and Metabolic Disorders?" *Molecular Nutrition and Food Research 58*(3): 537–549.

Scholey, A., A. Gibbs, C. Neale et al. 2014. "Anti-Stress Effects of Lemon Balm-Containing Foods." *Nutrients 6*(11): 4805–4821.

Sharma, V. K., M. Trakroo, V. Subramaniam et al. 2013. "Effect of Fast and Slow Pranayama on Perceived Stress and Cardiovascular

Parameters in Young Health-Care Students." *International Journal of Yoga 6*(2): 104–110.

Sirois, F. M., R. Kitner, and J. K. Hirsch. 2014. "Self-Compassion, Affect, and Health-Promoting Behaviors." *Health Psychology*. Advance online publication. Retrieved from http://dx.doi.org/10.1037/hea0000158.

Slayton, S. C., J. D'Archer, and F. Kaplan. 2010 "Outcome Studies on the Efficacy of Art Therapy: A Review of Findings." *Art Therapy: Journal of the American Art Therapy Association 27*(3): 108–118.

Song, C., H. Ikei, and Y. Miyazaki. 2014. "Elucidation of the Physiological Adjustment Effect of Forest Therapy." *Nihon Eiseigaku Zasshi 69*(2): 111–116.

Spence, C., and O. Deroy. 2013. "On Why Music Changes What (We Think) We Taste." *i-perception 16* 4(2): 137–140.

Stapleton, P., D. Church, T. Sheldon et al. 2013. "Depression Symptoms Improve after Successful Weight Loss with Emotional Freedom Techniques." *ISRN Psychiatry 2013* (2090–7966): 1–7. doi:10.1155/2013/573532.

Stewart, P., and E. Goss. 2013. "Plate Shape and Colour Interact to Influence Taste and Quality Judgments." *Flavour 2*(27).

Strassel, J. K., D. C. Cherkin, L. Steuten et al. 2011. "A Systematic Review of the Evidence for the Effectiveness of Dance Therapy." *Alternative Therapy Health Medicine 17*(3): 50–59.

Szekeres, R. A., and E. H. Wertheim. 2014. "Evaluation of Vipassana Meditation Course Effects on Subjective Stress, Well-Being, Self-Kindness and Mindfulness in a Community Sample: Post-Course and 6-Month Outcomes." *Stress and Health*. Advance online publication. doi:10.1002/smi.2562.

Taylor, H. A., and T. Tenbrink. 2013. "The Spatial Thinking of Origami: Evidence from Think-Aloud Protocols." *Cognitive Processing 14*(2): 189–191.

Telles, S., K. Maharana, B. Balrana et al. 2011. "Effects of High-Frequency Yoga Breathing Called *Kapalabhati* Compared with Breath Awareness on the Degree of Optical Illusion Perceived." *Perceptual and Motor Skills 112*(3): 981–990.

Telles, S., S. K. Sharma, and A. Balkrishna. 2014. "Blood Pressure and Heart Rate Variability During Yoga-Based Alternate Nostril Breathing Practice and Breath Awareness." *Medical Science Monitor Basic Research 19*(20): 184–193.

Teufel, M., K. Stephan, A. Kowalski et al. 2013. "Impact of Biofeedback on Self-Efficacy and Stress Reduction in Obesity: A Randomized Controlled Pilot Study." *Applied Psychophysiology Biofeedback 38*(3): 177–184.

Thoma, M. V., R. La Marca, R. Brönnimann et al. 2013. "The Effect of Music on the Human Stress Response." *PLoS One 8*(8): e70156.

Troisi, J. D., and S. Gabriel. 2011. "Chicken Soup Really Is Good for the Soul: 'Comfort Food' Fulfills the Need to Belong." *Psychological Science 22*(6): 747–753.

Turankar, A. V., S. Jain, S. B. Patel et al. 2013. "Effects of Slow Breathing Exercise on Cardiovascular Functions, Pulmonary Functions & Galvanic Skin Resistance in Healthy Human Volunteers: A Pilot Study." *Indian Journal of Medical Research 137*(5): 916–921.

van der Wal, R. C., and L. F. van Dillen. 2013. "Leaving a Flat Taste in Your Mouth: Task Load Reduces Taste Perception." *Psychological Science 24*(7): 1277–1284.

Van Oudenhove, L., S. McKie, D. Lassman et al. 2011. "Fatty Acid–Induced Gut-Brain Signaling Attenuates Neural and Behavioral Effects of Sad Emotion in Humans." *Journal of Clinical Investigation 121*(8): 3094–3099.

Vohs, K. D., Y. Wang, F. Gino et al. 2013. "Rituals Enhance Consumption." *Psychological Science 24*(9): 1714–1721.

Wang, H. P., J. Yang, L. Qin et al. 2015. "Effect of Garlic on Blood Pressure: A Meta-Analysis." *Journal of Clinical Hypertension 17*(3): 223–231.

Wansink, B., M. M. Cheney, and N. Chan. 2003. "Exploring Comfort Food Preferences across Age and Gender." *Physiology & Behavior 79*: 739–747.

Wansink, B., K. M. Kniffin, and M. Shimizu. 2012. "Death Row Nutrition: Curious Conclusions of Last Meals." *Appetite 59*(3): 837–843.

Wansink, B., and K. van Ittersum. 2012. "Fast Food Restaurant Lighting and Music Can Reduce Calorie Intake and Increase Satisfaction." *Psychological Reports: Human Resources & Marketing, 111*(1): 228–232.

Weltens, N., D. Zhao, and L. Van Oudenhove. 2014. "Where Is the Comfort in Comfort Foods? Mechanisms Linking Fat Signaling, Reward, and Emotion." *Neurogastroenterology & Motility 26*(3): 303–315.

Wood, A. M., S. Joseph, J. Lloyd et al. 2009. "Gratitude Influences Sleep Through the Mechanism of Pre-Sleep Cognitions." *Journal of Psychosomatic Research 66*(1): 43–48.

Yeo, S., K. S. Kim, and S. Lim. 2013. "Randomized Clinical Trial of Five Ear Acupuncture Points for the Treatment of Overweight People." *Acupuncture in Medicine 32*(2): 132–138.

Yoto, A., S. Murao, Y. Nakamura et al. 2014. "Intake of Green Tea Inhibited Increase of Salivary Chromogranin A After Mental Task Stress Loads." *Journal of Physiological Anthropology 33*(1): 20.

Young, S. N. 2007. "How to Increase Serotonin in the Human Brain Without Drugs." *Journal of Psychiatry & Neuroscience 32*(6): 394–399.

Zoccola, P. M., W. S. Figueroa, E. M. Rabideau et al. 2014. "Differential Effects of Poststressor Rumination and Distraction on Cortisol and C-Reactive Protein." *Health Psychology 33*(12): 1606–1609.

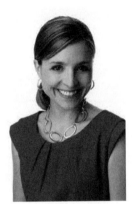

Photo by Martha Stutzman

Susan Albers, PsyD, is a psychologist at the Cleveland Clinic who specializes in eating issues, weight loss, body image concerns, and mindfulness. Albers conducts mindful eating workshops across the country, and is a frequent keynote speaker. She is author of seven mindful eating books, including the *New York Times* bestseller *Eat Q*; *50 Ways to Soothe Yourself Without Food*; *But I Deserve This Chocolate!*; *Eating Mindfully*; *Eat, Drink, and Be Mindful*; and *Mindful Eating 101*. Her work has been featured in *O*, *Family Circle*, *Shape*, *Prevention*, *Self*, *Health*, *Fitness*, *Vanity Fair*, *Natural Health*, and *The Wall Street Journal*. She has been a guest on *The Dr. Oz Show*, and is also a contributor to *The Huffington Post* and *Psychology Today*.

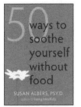
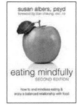
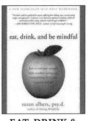
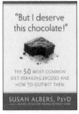

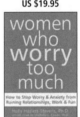